WHEN

THE WOLF

IS AT THE

DOOR

WHEN
THE WOLF
IS AT THE
DOOR

The Simplicity
of HEALING

by Michele Longo O'Donnell

LA VIDA PRESS
BOERNE, TX

ISBN 978-0-9814649-1-6 hardcover
ISBN 978-0-9814649-0-9 softcover

Published in 2007 by
La Vida Press
107 Scenic Loop Rd
Boerne, TX 78006
830-755-8767

Cover design and illustration by Travis Ward

Printed in USA

To Peggy and Ray
You are the deepest motivation in my soul.
One day mankind will know and accept...
and everything will be different.

TABLE OF CONTENTS

"And I heard a great voice out of heaven saying, Behold, the tabernacle of God is with men, and he will dwell with them, and they shall be his people and God himself shall be with them, for he is their (Life) God.

And God shall wipe away all tears from their eyes; and there shall be no more death, neither shall there be any more pain; for the former things are passed away.

....Behold, I make all things new."

Revelation 21:3-5

❧

"That thou may love the Lord thy God, and that thou may obey His voice, and that thou may cleave unto Him: *for He is thy Life* and the length of thy days."

Deuteronomy 30:20

PREFACE

The simplicity of healing? How can that possibly be? Healing has been anything but simple. The quest for healing has been the most sought after, complicated, convoluted, protracted and illusive endeavor of mankind for as long as history has been recorded. But I have come to think that instead of wondering why it is simple, we ought to be wondering why it has been made to be so impossible.

Could it be because we were unaware that we were meant to be able to heal whatever appeared that threatened to harm us? Could it be because we believed that disease came from something wrong within us and not as we now know... simply as a suggestion of evil, a suggestion of an ability to interrupt something God has made? Before anything can reach us to manifest against us, we must first acquiesce to the lie that God's creation can be somehow interrupted, maligned. Once we have agreed to that we have become vulnerable to whatever comes to suggest itself a power other than God. A power greater than and able to overcome and destroy the works of God.

I now see all disease as an interruption in the intact and eternal state of perfection in which we are formed. But since His works are uninterruptible, we must have first surrendered to many such beliefs in order for disease to reach us in the first place. "All the works of His hands are perfect." And, "It is He who has made us and not we ourselves." We first blindly accepted that we could experience it. Then we had to be made to believe we had no choice. We had to be convinced of our inherent weakness and vulnerability. We had to be made to feel we earned or deserved our fate. Somehow it is all our fault. We had to be made to believe we needed the suffering for a greater good. Many strange and convoluted ideologies were put into a pill for us to swallow...and as a whole human race...we swallowed it all!

Just as the experience of disease began with a thought, a belief, an acceptance of many things untrue, so the healing of it must begin with another thought, another perception which will realistically negate the first. We must understand once again who we are, where we have come from, why we are here and in what condition we have been made. We must reclaim our authority and sense of dominion. We must lose the victim mentality and stand on our feet as the eternal, mighty Sons of God that we are.

A lady recently healed of ovarian cancer made this bold and time arresting statement to me. She said, "My change came when I realized I had a choice!" You see first we have been lulled into a stupor of resignation to disease as a power greater than God, greater than ourselves. Then we have been taught that we must deal with it on the same level that it appeared...strictly physical. So we subject our bodies to mutilating surgeries, pathogenic toxic drugs, and myriads of "diagnostic" gyrations. As we sacrifice our bodies upon the alter of modern science, have we realized that we are not getting better but instead much sicker as a whole? We have not found what we seek because we are looking in the wrong direction, digging the hole deeper and deeper.

Healing becomes so simple once we turn from all this madness and choose to look long and hard at the Glory and Light which lies within us. "For of His fullness have we all received." We find that healing is not something that must happen from outside of ourselves, but instead is an unlocking of something so powerful, so available and so easily released from within each one...no matter who we are or what weird roads we have traveled. "For we have this treasure in earthen vessels, that the Excellency of the power may be of God and not of ourselves."

Nothing new needs to be added, sought after or discovered. Only released. Only revealed. We don't need a miracle. We only need to find how easily we can allow the intrinsic wholeness, which is the natural state of our existence, to be freed. One paradigm shift of thought, of true understanding, will correct all conditions of confusion and darkness we call dis-ease. The beloved American poet, Robert Browning referred to this as the "release of the imprisoned Splendor."

There is a path of freedom, of release, and it is as near to each one as the breath we breathe. The way is clear, simple and easily obtainable. I used to think that there was no clear "formula" for healing, but in a way there is. I hope to have captured for you this understanding in these pages. Suffering is such an unnecessary human experience. The real tragedy lies in that we so readily accept it.

This is the third book in a trilogy called Living Beyond Disease. If you haven't read the first two, you might want to start there for a continuity of understanding.

INTRODUCTION

Why do some people who really embrace and love the truth still fail in healing themselves or others? Isn't it true that the truth shall make us free? Isn't the truth true? If so, how can we miss?

Recently I knew of a lady who was in this situation. She found herself facing a threatening illness and yet for all her past experience of healing so many others, she, herself, failed to heal. I was perplexed, to say the least, and so I did what I always do when I am perplexed...I sought the Mind of Wisdom for my answers.

All my life people have asked me how am I able to heal...especially during those early years when I was so steeped in traditional religion and totally unaware of the deeper truths of God. And I always gave them the patented answer, "I don't heal, God does." I knew my singular response was shallow and really not answering what they were asking in their hearts. But I didn't even know myself why or how for a very long time. When the answer finally came,

I understood.

In John's first letter or epistle, he writes of a spiritual union or marriage, so to speak, between the truth (word) and the Spirit. He tells us that this union, deep within our souls, is necessary in order to live the life of the Son of God...including the healings we were sent to do. He said that the truth and Spirit "bear witness one to the other." The equation is incomplete without these two in agreement...or congruent.

I began my Spiritual life in a non-denominational Charismatic, Holy Ghost, "rompin, stompin" Church. Later I was ordained in an Assembly of God, or Pentecostal Church. I was deeply entrenched in the moving of the Spirit of God. I was familiar with listening to Its voice for direction and Wisdom. I was thoroughly convinced of my own inadequacies without this direction… in every aspect of my life. The focus was to "Love the Lord, God with all our hearts, minds, strength and hearts." And I did and I do. My basic foundation was a relationship of love and trust. It was personal and deeply felt. This is being in a state of oneness with the Spirit of God. A marriage or a union with Spirit.

From there I was introduced to the deeper truths of the Kingdom of God. My heart cried out for relief from suffering for the world, children in specific, and I ached to understand why this misery continued, even for those who knew God in the same way that I did.

My prayers and my search found me hearing of our basic "oneness" with God, what Jesus prayed we would come to know in John 17. I came to understand that there really was only OneLife and that was the Life of God. That everything created was an expression of His life and as we yielded to this we would realize the truth of it. I began to understand that we live by what is eternally true and not by what we are seeing or experiencing. I found that these things would be corrected as folks embraced their basic union and oneness with God as their Life. Not something to achieve but to accept. All things were done, finished and complete. Our problem was that we didn't know or believe that. We were convinced that we were here to achieve, to earn that fullness...not that we came only to express it...as that fullness (John 1) "Of His fullness have we all received." This is being in a state of oneness with the Spirit of truth. A marriage or union with truth.

These truths were always right there in my beloved Scriptures...but I never saw them before. I was blinded by what I was being taught. It took quite a number of dedicated years to unlearn a lot of what I had heard, but I finally was able to sort it all out. What never changed was my love for God, my devotion to Jesus and my absolute trust in the guidance and direction, counsel and Wisdom of Spirit as I yielded to it.

This then was the union, the marriage in my soul. I received the best from both (religious) worlds, so to speak: The Spirit and the truth. Truthfully, I ache for those two worlds to come together as I have done. They each bring such absolutes, both sides of the necessary equation for fullness.

All too often I see folks who are well versed in truth have a relationship with the truth instead of the truth-giver.

It seems the love, the devotion, the commitment to God's purpose for their existence (instead of their own) has been supplanted by a teaching of self-serving, self-attaining. Love implies a whole hearted devotion to another...no matter what the personal cost to oneself. This is what Jesus taught, this is what he lived and this is why he was able to do the things he did.

At the same time Jesus taught us who we really are and that we were to embrace that in humility and obedience to the greater purpose. He taught the true nature of God to man, and the true nature of man in God... which has been swallowed up in the doctrines and traditions of men.

So the two are necessary to complete the whole. One without the other is only half of the picture. We should learn from one another. We lose when we judge and turn away from others. Each part of the whole is so necessary to the total whole.

"Those who are led by the Spirit of God shall be called the Sons of God."

Those who are led by the traditions and doctrines, fads and fashions, they only hear... are as the "blind leading the blind and they both fall into the ditch!"

We must open our hearts to God. The way into the Kingdom is through the heart...never the intellect. Our lives are not our own, we come with a purpose and that is not our own either. This is the way to find the fullness we wish to experience. This is the way to healings and total restoration of all things.

May the eyes and hearts of all who read this be opened

and filled with the Spirit of God, the Spirit of Love and the Spirit of Truth. Amen.

.

CHAPTER ONE

WHEN THE WOLF IS AT THE DOOR

In my second book, "The God That We've Created, The Basic Cause of all Disease," I told the story of my healing from cervical cancer. The method by which I was healed left an indelible mark on my soul, one of being loved, cherished and eternally cared for. Because this had such a profound effect on me, irrespective of the healing that followed, I dedicated the title of this book to the whole experience. I know we are encouraged to believe that "Nothing shall by any means hurt you." But so often we struggle with that truth when faced with an alarming threat to our welfare. What I received from Divine Love Itself was of such great significance during that time, I would pray for everyone to experience it as well. Never again is there a need for a "prayer for protection." Never again is there a threat so viable as to make me feel less than forever safe and secure in the arms of Love. This feeling and surety of Love's love for us, in us and through us is so profoundly needed for permanent healings that I would like once again to share this story with you. Hopefully this will catapult you also into a world without disease, risk or threat.

Not long ago I was accompanying my youngest daughter to one of her pre-natal visits. I was anxious to meet her OB doctor, having heard so many nice things about him from her. During the visit his assistant discovered that I had never submitted to a test for cervical cancer. Actually, I had never been to a doctor for any tests or check-ups since my babies were born and had no thought to do so. But for a reason unknown to me at the time I decided to let the test be done that day. I left and returned home, thinking nothing of it again. A few days later I received a call from the doctor's office saying that the test was positive for cervical cancer. They told me that the abnormal cells were quite extensive throughout the cervix and I should come in immediately to talk with the doctor.

Once I realized what was being said to me, I quickly shifted into the spiritual mode of thought. Since I was convinced that I was a child of Light, sent to "undo the works of darkness," and "nothing shall by any means hurt me," I concluded that this was simply an evidence of darkness that needed to be dissolved by the shining of the light of truth. I told the nurse that I would not do anything until after my granddaughter was born. This was a very special and sacred time for our family and I wasn't going to allow evil in any shape or form to spoil it. This also was my way of putting her off until I had the chance to pray about the whole thing. Two of my assistants at the clinic, and very dear friends, were standing beside me when the call came in. I asked them to support me in prayer and not say a word to anyone, not even to speak of this between themselves. They agreed. We are quite cognizant of the power of our words for good or ill, so this was not foreign to them. I determined not to tell anyone in my family either until I had a chance to pray about it, which was pretty much how I always handle problems anyway. The more people who know about specific challenges, the more their fears and concerns cloud up the 'atmosphere of thought,' making extrication from any situation more difficult.

One month later my daughter gave birth to her baby and we were able to rejoice, enjoying every moment of the experience without any gloom hanging over us. Soon we all settled back into our life routines and I began to ask God to prepare space for me to deal with this now.

During my daughter's first post natal visit to her doctor's office, the nurse told her what was going on with me, with the hope that she would have some influence to convince me to return to them for treatment. So now the whole family knew. I agreed to a biopsy where the performing physician described in detail the "masses" that he observed and the 'salt and pepper' scatterings of abnormal cells throughout.

We returned home where we began to quietly, but fervently pray. I began to feel the strength of their support and knew it was time to 'press in.' The whole effort took about three days. The house was quiet, the atmosphere was focused, but confident. I stayed awake all night the first night, reading and remembering who I am, why I have come here and simply feeling the Presence of Divine Love. This enabled me to gain entrance into the "Sabbath rest," which I knew would allow space for God to speak. This entering into the "rest" allowed all anxiety to subside, and the realization of Love began to fill my heart.

This challenge came after years of studying, questioning, learning and seeing thousands of irrefutable proofs of the truths I was being taught. I determined to allow this temple of my soul to be filled with the Presence and Power of the Glory of God. It replaced the lingering unrest, fear and dread, and total distortion of truth, that the dark suggestions of the human consciousness always carries.

My foundation of thought began with remembering what I already knew to be true, setting the cornerstone for the Holy Spirit to begin to build whatever new understandings it would.

I remembered that I am a child of Light, not a result of a random DNA, nor the will of my parents.

I remembered that I was not dealing with disease. But instead, I was dealing with Divine Love, for Love is Omnipresent...the knowledge of which cancels any place or space for evil to exist.

I remembered that I was sent to this earthly existence, not to seek my own self interests, not to preserve this mortal experience, but to fulfill the purpose of God. And to let the expression of truth, harmony and perfection have the freedom to appear in any given situation.

I remembered that my life is 'not my own.' I do not have an individual life, separate and apart from the One Life that is God...or the one expression of that Life, which is called the Christ. ("When Christ, *who is your life* shall appear..")

I remembered that the reason we, as the light, have appeared in this earthly form was to 'undo the works of darkness'... and how could we do this unless we come face to face with it?

I remembered that the will and purpose of God is to reveal His Glory. That is, to appear as the Light, harmony, beauty and perfection to every appearance of darkness.

I remembered that this was really not about me at all! Knowing all this with all my heart, I was able to surrender to the grace that I knew must flow through my soul and my mind, for only by grace, the activity of Spirit, would this darkness be resolved and the light of the Glory of God be revealed.

The next morning I received a call from Kay, one of the two friends who stood beside me when I first received the news. She also had been praying and during this time heard a word over and over again in her mind, giving her impulse to look up the definition in the dictionary. The word was "disdain." The first definition was the common one, "to look at someone with condescending contempt, from an ignoble mind." But the second listed definition was what prompted her to call me. It said, "A passionate, forceful hatred of evil from a noble mind." We both realized that this was declaring that the Christ, (the Spirit of God revealed through creation) stood before this evil, not only in our behalf, but in behalf of the appearing of the harmony and perfection of God, replacing the human beliefs with the Divine Mind. In other words, God was already "on it!"

Evil loves to declare its right to exist, to be feared and honored as a power to contend with. It loves to usurp its authority over the authority of Eternal Life and immense Love. It declares darkness to be stronger than light, hate to be stronger than love, confusion to be stronger than order, lies to be stronger than truth. But here was the Christ, declaring its Power, its Presence, its authority, its truth.

When I heard those words, I felt a definite shift in consciousness and realized that I had once again entered into the "rest" of the Sabbath. Peace and assurance flooded my soul. I felt an overwhelming sense of gratitude and knew I would be "led" as to what I should do, if anything. I knew that no matter what I must face, I was going to be okay. Everything was going to be okay!

The next day while at the clinic, I was climbing into the chamber of the hyperbaric oxygen unit to arrange something for a patient when I suddenly had a very definite and intense vision of a wolf standing before me, fierce and aggressive, with its eyes yellow and slanted, baring its teeth. This animal was in "attack mode!" Instantly the form of a shepherd jumped between us. Facing the wolf, I could see the back of his robe-like garment with a rope tied about his waist. His legs were spread, his arms raised and a cat-o'-nine-tails whip was in his right hand. He was defending his lamb. It all happened so fast when I heard the words, "The wolf is at the door." I immediately responded, "I know!" "But don't worry, Michele," I heard him say. "I am the door"

With those words the vision vanished. Melissa, the other friend who was with me at the first phone call, was also in the chamber behind me. I turned to her and collapsed, stunned and in tears I kept repeating, "Melissa, the wolf is at the door, but He is the door!" Over and over again I said those words, crying so hard she could barely understand me. I had never felt such love in all my life. Patiently she sat with me, not knowing what could have prompted this sudden emotion, and held my hand until the impact of the whole experience began to subside. I was telling her the vision when the phone rang. It was the doctor's office with the report from the biopsy. I cannot tell you how peaceful I was taking that phone call. It may as well have been a weather report! They told me what I expected to hear, there was no sign, no observable indication of anything wrong at all. Later I asked the doctor what he thought of it all. He had just finished reading my first book, "Of Monkeys and Dragons, Freedom from the Tyranny of Disease," so he smiled and said, "I would have expected nothing less!"

This is the result of knowing the truth, of entering into the "rest" of God, which comes from *believing* what you have come to know as truth. This is the clear result of the free flow of grace fulfilling the will of God, and bringing harmony to every human event. It is available for everyone right now, it is the reason that we exist here in this human form.

Once again I must say that the love and assurance, confidence and unusual feeling of immortality that flooded my soul with those words and the subsequent healing that followed, has eternally impacted my entire existence. I carry it into every situation I am asked to pray about. This love, this being so cared for and cherished is for every person, every animal, everything created. It is for us all and in us all. Robert Browning, the eloquent poet, spoke of this as "The Imprisoned Splendor." It only needs to be allowed to be released into expression.

CHAPTER TWO

THE KEY TO THE KINGDOM

I want to start out by saying that when you really actively realize the depth of God's love for you, you will be healed.

We measure that love by how much we think our parents loved us, our spouses love us, our friends and children love us. We have an image of our selves and if we, by our standards, measure up to that image, then we think we are loved. It's crazy but we all fall into that. If we don't measure up, then we are not loved.

So I hear all the time, "I think that I am not doing something right." This invokes fear in the heart, thinking that if I don't get it right I might not get this healing that I so desperately need. Who said that God was waiting for us to do anything anyway? What makes us think that we must qualify for His Love or care? We are His creation. We are His offspring. We are His sheep and He is responsible for us. "It is He who made us and not we ourselves." It is He who makes the seasons change. It is He who feeds the roaming animals. It is He who makes the world turn. "He opens his hand and satisfies the desire of every living thing."

All we need to do is give Him full reign. And we have not done this because we have been told that He might hurt us, or "allow" us to be hurt, (for our own good, of course.) We've been told that He might hurt us either because we failed, or because we need to suffer for whatever might be gained by doing so.

Therefore we are afraid to trust Him with this life we call ours. But really our lives belong to God from beginning to end. He formed us. He sent us. He has purpose in doing this. He decides the purpose, forms us, sends us, and then it is He who performs whatever we were sent to do. Hear the words of Job. "He performs that thing which is appointed for me to do."

We fall apart because we are holding on so tightly. We are making decisions, drawing upon our own limited resources, trusting in our efforts to get this life lived. We draw from the wisdom of man which is no wisdom at all...just opinions. If we want real substantial Wisdom, Eternal, forever lasting Wisdom which will always mean goodness and Life, we must let go of the hold and give this life...which is His to start with... back to him and CHOOSE to trust.

To help us know how much we are loved, Jesus uses the example of God as our Shepherd and we as His sheep. Now sheep don't know their right hand from their left and depend completely upon their Shepherd for their very existence. So it ought to be with us. We will never know how good it can be until we surrender to Him...even if we are terrified to do it at first.

Jesus said, "Fear not little flock, it is your Father's good pleasure to give you the Kingdom." He said that God's Love is such that He would leave 99 sheep to go out and find the one who is lost. He instructed Peter at the shores of Galilee to "Feed my sheep."

Some of you may remember the song, "I surrender all." If I have sung that once, I have sung it a thousand times in my life. I want God to know, I want my soul to know, I want the whole of Eternity to know that I do not consider my life to be my own but it belongs to Him who made it and sent it with purpose. I want to be that sheep who follows closely beside the Shepherd's tent and knows every beat of His heart, so I can stay tuned in all the time. I want to always feel loved and cared for. I want this life to count for something more than my own selfish needs fulfilled. I want to hear at the end of this time, "Well done my good and faithful servant."

If we do not know this Love of God for us, we must ask to know it. We must ask and ask for the grace to trust Him who loves us. We must know it will be better, much better for us when we choose to trust. We must stop trying to do everything right, we must stop trying, period, and just rest in His care.

CHAPTER THREE

THE POWER OF SURRENDER

From the time we are first introduced to the "ways of God" we hear the instruction to "surrender" whenever we are facing a difficult situation. If you are anything like me you have probably struggled with that one. Why must we surrender? What are we surrendering to? How does this help, or does it help at all? Surrendering seems so frightening to most of us and confusing as well. Nevertheless, it is the only way. So let's explore it together.

Jesus, as our example, surrendered his whole life, every moment, every decision, every thought. It was in this surrendering that he found his Wisdom, his power, his strength for every situation and to fulfill his Father's purpose for his life. He described this necessary attitude of the heart when he said, "To gain your Life, you must be willing to lose your life. He who would save his life will lose it and he who is willing to lose his life will save it." The act of losing your life does not mean physically dying but "dying to the self-life." Dying to your present identity as a vulnerable mortal with a variety of desires, needs and demands. *Letting go of your present image of your life in favor of the true image that God holds in His Mind of your Life.* In other words, acknowledge that your Life is not your own! But your Life is God's Eternal Life, for there is but One Life. So, now, how does this play out in daily living? It means that He makes the decisions, He makes the way. It is His Wisdom, His counsel, His direction we yield to and not our own way, our own means, our own solutions. This is what it means to "lose your life." Lose your control. Lose your will. And take on the Father's will, the Father's purpose and intention and how Divine Wisdom wants any given thing done.

Scary? Only if you don't really "know" God. If there is any hint of the "old image of God" left, this idea will scare you. To surrender control you must trust God...trust Love...trust Wisdom. You will never be able to trust God while yet holding onto the old idea of God...one that makes God responsible for your pain and loss. If you don't realize God as Mercy Itself, if you don't realize that God is always for you and never against you, if you have any notion that you might have deserved this misery...in all this you will freeze up when it comes to surrendering.

Just in case I might have inadvertently "drawn this problem"...because there is this mortal law of reaping what you have sown... I always begin my prayer by repenting for anything I may have thought, believed, said or done that was contrary to my true nature. *Once I do that I know it no longer has any affect upon me at all.* I am that convinced of God's goodness and Mercy and I am that convinced of my true nature as His image, His visible manifestation on the earth. Therefore my sincere act of repentance completely eliminates the thought of having to suffer for past or present offense. Also I really work on being merciful. That I may "be my Father's representative," (who is Mercy Itself) and that I may obtain Mercy when I so frequently need it.

Romans 8 declares that the law of attraction is eliminated by the Law of the Spirit of Life. "For the Law of the Spirit of Life has made me free from the law of sin and death." *The Law of the Spirit of Life is a declaration that you know and have fully embraced; there is but One Life, it is God, and you are a visible manifestation of that One Life.* Therefore you are above and out of reach of any "lesser" mortal law, such as the law of sowing and reaping. Yes, it says, "God is not mocked, whatsoever you sow, that shall you also reap." But this only holds true of the old image of mortal frailty. Now that you are a "new creature" in Christ Jesus, (hid in the Life and Spirit of Jesus Christ), "all the old has passed away and all things are new." (11Corinthians, chapter 5) This is the value of sincere repentance. It reminds us who we really are when we so often forget. It is the greatest tool we have for making the "inside of the cup clean." The Prophet, Daniel prayed three times a day, repenting for his transgressions, thus keeping the soul clean and a ready conduit for the flow of the Spirit of life. This devotion and habit of prayer came in handy when facing the hungry lions and will likewise come in handy for you in the hour you may have to face your "lions."

Once that is done, all that is left in my whole thought is receiving Wisdom and council for whatever I face. We must know what is the ultimate purpose and intention of God. We cannot be hazy about this or we will fail to trust. God's intention is to demonstrate that *the Kingdom of God is here and now, present and available on earth as it is in Heaven.* This was Jesus' whole ministry. He healed, he fed, he spoke and he rose from the dead, all to demonstrate that the only power here is the Power of God (endless Life) and God is only good! He spoke incessantly about the immediate presence of the Kingdom of God, about the rule and reign of One Power, One God. *His definition of the Kingdom of God was living in the Presence, authority and dominion of Mercy and Love. He proved it was here by all he did.*

For centuries we have been robbed of this reality by those who declare that Heaven is something we must attain to and we do this after we die and by suffering here on earth. Jesus said the Kingdom of Heaven is within you right here, right now. Paul said that in this "we live and move and have our being." We are "In Him," as spoken throughout and He is in the Kingdom of God...actually He IS the Kingdom of God!

Understanding this will enable you to surrender *quickly* to Eternal Wisdom *without trying to hold onto the outcome.* It will enable you to immediately trust and then patiently wait for the harmony and goodness to appear. Without this understanding, you may *finally* surrender (and then find appearing what you desired in the first place,) but it will be with much pain and effort before getting to this.

Early in the course of my life I held onto things for years, praying, crying and dragging out the problem because I was too ignorant or afraid to "let it go and trust it with God." I thought that if I let it go, it may never come back. Finally I had to let it go because it was killing me to hang on. And in each situation, the Light would break forth and goodness would appear in such abundance and such beauty...beyond what I had been telling God or begging God to do. Until I ceased from my outlining 'what and how,' until I finally 'let it go' to God's will, I was paralyzed. Only after years of struggles and hundreds of times of finally surrendering...and then seeing the consistency of the goodness that followed...did I began to trust. I began to know God. I began to understand that it was always the intention of God to do "exceedingly abundantly above all that I could ask or think." It is always God's intention to reveal the Power of His kingdom, His absolute ruling authority.

Remember, and this is really important, you are not surrendering to the disease, the division, the loss, the lack or any other suggestion of evil! You are only and always surrendering to the absolute, unchangeable, Nature of God. And God is, above all else, Mercy. And God wants, above all else, the establishment of His Kingdom here on earth. He wants to demonstrate His glorious Nature in, to and through us all. You are surrendering to the Power of God only!

You see, evil suggestions come to declare *one thing only*. No matter how evil appears, in what form or event...it always declares that it is a power. That it has the Power of God. That it has the ability to hurt or to destroy. Never mind that you are the Holy Son of God and that "no evil can come nigh your dwelling place!" Never mind that you are "hid in Christ in God." Nothing can touch you! Never mind that God has never created a power apart from Himself, nor has He ever used His Power to hurt or harm...that would be against His own Nature to do so. "He cannot deny Himself."

In every situation presented to man by the darkness of the human mind, evil will tell you it has the power to destroy you. It may tell you that God, Himself sent it to "wake you up, to punish you, to direct you." It will tell you a lot of things, but if you know what is true you can tell it a thing or two! As you stand facing it fearlessly, *your words are the power of God.* Watch it run! "The weapons of our warfare are not carnal (human means) but they are spiritual, unto the pulling down of strongholds (of the mind)."

Every situation is an opportunity to declare... and know... that there is only One Power. Actually this is the whole spiritual battle. No matter how it presents, it is *just darkness* declaring itself a power and you standing there deciding if that is true or not. If you are terrorized by it, you are declaring you agree with it...that it is a power to destroy. If you stand facing it with the word and truth and strength of *knowing* God as the One and only Power, you will see the "goodness of God in the land of the living!' It is NEVER about what has appeared. No matter how obtrusive the appearance may be. It is *always* about "where is the power!" If we get caught up in trying to fix the problem, we are still declaring it is a power to contend with. If we turn immediately to face the Glory of God in His Kingdom... right here, right now, no matter what else is appearing...we will be agreeing with God and allowing that Power to flow.

It is not a battle between "good and evil" as the world declares. That would be agreeing that evil is indeed a power, and it isn't! It is a battle of faith...of what we are believing. Of where we place the power and authority. "Therefore, fight the good fight of faith." Nowhere does it say to fight against anything or anyone!

But if you are wringing your hands, pacing and worrying....if you cannot surrender it to God...you are declaring that you don't know or trust God. You can and must quickly repent of this thought, pray for the grace to realize and hold to God as the only Power here, and then let Him do the rest for you. *Don't try to make yourself believe what you can't.* Just repent for what you *are* believing, ask for the grace to see it differently, and I promise God will take it from there.

If you are still under the delusion that you are living "your life," you are not! If you think this is your life and you are personally responsible for it, you are not! There is only *One Life* and that Life is God and we live it by letting Him live it *as us, through us.* We possess nothing. We are responsible for nothing...except to surrender to His will and to love one another. "For of Him and through Him and to Him are all things."

The whole nature of God, the whole purpose of God and all the promises of God, are instantly activated as soon as we surrender to Him...declaring we trust Him, we belong to Him and our Life is not our own!

❧

It is not *God* who needs us to surrender. It is *we* who need to surrender. This moves away all blocks, all obstructions, all hindrances to the free flow of the Eternal Spirit of God and allows Life to appear.

In Ezekiel, chapter 44, we read that the priests could not approach God wearing anything that "causes them to sweat." This is signifying that we must not yield to human labor, effort or personal responsibility, but yield to the Wisdom, counsel and purpose of God as soon as possible when darkness/ evil suggests its ugly words and threats against us.

When ever "lack or limitation, disease, or division" comes knocking on our door declaring it can take from us, think on this. What do we have that was not given to us by the Father? Then what can evil take? Would it not be taking from God only? Can it take from God?

The first time I was told to surrender to God I balked. But then I heard, "What do you have to loose? Haven't you lost everything already?" And so I had! Surrendering gave me back my life…in spades!

Stop, wait, ask for Wisdom and counsel, release it to the Power of God and then SING! Sing with your whole heart. You magnify the Power of God when you sing to Him and about Him. You let that Spirit fill your whole mind and heart and nothing, absolutely nothing of confusion or pain can remain in there when it is filled with song. How would you feel if the problem, the threat wasn't there? Act as though it already isn't there. In the Mind of God, it isn't!

CHAPTER FOUR

FOOTSTEPS TO HEALING

What should we do or think when faced with a problem? Every problem is a temptation to believe in a power other than God, who produces only goodness. It is a temptation to believe that something can interrupt the uninterruptible...which is the creation of God, for His creation is a *manifestation of Himself.*

So the first thing to do is to ask yourself, "Am I fearful, angry, or disturbed by this in any way?" If the answer is "yes," then repent quickly for giving it power, when clearly it is no power at all. It may boast of being a power. It may point out all the destruction it has done to others. (But remember that they had to have believed in its ability to do so.) It may try to scare you to death with all its declarations of greatness...but one moment of repentance will shut it up. Don't try to fight against it. You then are declaring that it is a power to fight against. Don't resist it head on at all. Just turn to face the unmovable Presence of the Power and Glory of God and repent for any power you have agreed to...

other than Him. Immediately you will feel a release. If you are afraid, it will subside. If you are in pain it will leave you. If you are paralyzed by fear, you will feel a growing peacefulness and confidence. All because you rejected it. All because you released it from your soul thereby *making space* for grace to fill your entire being.

If it comes back, and it very well may, just do it again. Tell it to leave. Tell it who you are and who has the power here! Tell it that it is an *unwelcome intruder* in your life (which is really God's Life) and that it has no business bothering you. You will be amazed at the immediate results. Just stay with it as long as you need to. Don't be "weary in well doing, for after you have done what God requires of you, you SHALL obtain the promise."

There are amazing doctrines going around these days which seem to be dazzling the masses. They sound so good but fail to deliver the desired results. Unless you have been grounded in truth you will find you have been mesmerized yourself by some of these.

One is that your own thoughts have brought this grief upon you. You are the Son of God. "For the Spirit of Christ dwells in you!" There is only One Son of God and we are all *in Him*. One in Him.

You have the Mind of Christ. There is only One Mind and you possess it. You cannot think or know anything other than what God thinks and knows. If it seems that you have, it is only *world thought* that has attached itself to you. Your thought, your understanding, is still and always intact...eternally. But as we walk through this *maze of con-*

fusion of thought, much seems to attach itself to us like dust does to our feet. Choosing to think the true thoughts out from the Mind that is God, thereby replacing the negative, intruding thoughts, is like washing away the dust from our feet. Jesus said to Peter, when He was washing his feet at the Last Supper, "If I wash your feet, you are clean all over. You only have need that your feet be washed." Meaning that we are whole and complete and that is an immutable fact of Being and nothing can change that. But daily we need to wash our feet, so to speak, and also others as they desire us to, and the Present Perfection of the Divine Life becomes the only thing left to see.

So it is not "your thought, or their thought" which you are dealing with. It is simply *world* thought. You and they are perfect, whole and complete. You must not attach condemnation to yourself or another. We don't have the power to create evil. We don't create good either. We just *manifest* what God is, eternally. All the creating that needed to be done is finished...it only needs to be revealed now. And as we make space for that to happen, it will... with no effort and no resistance. NOTHING NEW NEEDS TO BE CREATED FOR ANYONE TO BE WELL. God is not recreating you or me. God is *revealing what lies within us*. It will surface as soon as we allow it to.

There is no condition that needs to be removed or circumstance that needs to be corrected. Only intruding thoughts which need to be sent away.

The second doctrine we have all heard is that affliction is a result of past sins which need to be punished. This is a hard one because we all know that there is a law governing the "natural man" called the law of sowing and reaping. "Whatsoever you sow, that also shall you reap." But there is another, a higher law in operation here. It is the "Law of the Spirit of the One Life!" When we realize and embrace the knowledge that there is One Life only and that we are a manifestation of that One Life, we cannot be affected by the first law. One voids or disannuls the other. "For the Law of the Spirit of Life has made me free from the law of sin and death."

The first law was put into effect to keep creation in order but only until each one comes to accept the truth of who he is and who he has always been. Once the Spirit of Truth begins to reveal the truth of the One Life to the individual heart, and we make a decision to yield to the will and purpose of that One Life, that then is the only Law functional.

King David realized this when he said, "Blessed is the man to whom the Lord does not impute iniquity." Sin belongs to a false sense of life. Sin, still active, will punish the sinner so long as he remains in the thought of being a vulnerable mortal. But once he is raised in consciousness to know God as the only Presence, the only Power, the only Being...and we all as manifestations of that One...we can say with Paul, "I am the righteousness of God in Christ!" Daniel says in Psalms, "If you, Lord, punish iniquity, who then shall stand?"

No! God see us and deals with us as He made us, pure, perfect, whole and complete. When, in the first chapter of Genesis, God looked upon all that He had made and declared it all to be *very good*...the word good here in the Hebrew translation actually means, *indestructible, uninterruptible, incorruptible and perfect.*

If this is what God sees, then this is what is. If this is what God sees then there would be no need to punish. It is in the realization of this that men cease to sin. Remember that it is the *"goodness of God* that leads men to repentance." Not punishment.

I will say this many times throughout this work because *when men cease to accept suffering from the hand of God, they will cease to experience it.* It will then be only an *intrusion* in life and can therefore be immediately rejected. But so long as men believe that they have somehow earned their suffering, or that they are not worthy to receive a healing...(same thing!)...they will remain in their pain.

It is so very critical to realize that suffering has no basis at all. You didn't cause it. God didn't cause it. The guy next door didn't cause it. No one caused anything! It is from beginning to end an *intrusion of thought.* The Bible calls it an "evil imagination!" Ecclesiastes says, "God made man to walk in authority and dominion and power, as a prince...but man has sought out many evil imaginations!" First we imagine, then we blame God, or ourselves, for the results of that imaging! Then we run around trying to find someone who can make the image go away!

Last summer my granddaughter was two years old. She is fair complected and has rather sensitive skin. She also attracts bug bites by the scores! We tried every salve, every lotion, everything out there to try to relieve her of the bug bites. One day her baby brother, who was one year old at the time, bit her on her shoulder. He was teething and used all of us to bite on. Finally their dad became exasperated with all the injuries from his biting and told him "No!" He must have said it with conviction because the biting stopped. A few days later I noticed that my granddaughter's ankle was black and swollen. She began to cry with pain as I scrambled around frantically to find something to relieve the obvious fire ant attack she had incurred. Evidently the incident with her brother really made an impression with her. She watched me running around to find help for her and finally said, "Grandma! Just say NO!"

Good grief! Why hadn't I thought of that! I stopped, laughed, picked her up and we both said, "NO! No more, never again!" We went to the back yard and said, "NO!" We went to the front yard and said, "NO!" As you might imagine, the pain stopped, the swelling and blackness disappeared. She reminded me of the obvious. " God gave us dominion over everything that creeps and crawls"...etc. And (again) "nothing shall by any means hurt you!"

A third and very popular doctrine which holds us in the consciousness of suffering is the one that says that we have, by suffering and dying, something far greater to gain. It speaks of a Heaven far away and unattainable except by suffering. It gives us the notion that we must earn this place. And therefore we could easily fail to earn it. It does not tell us that we are in it now and always have been. "For in Him we live and move and have our being... and we are NOW "seated at the right hand of the Father, all power and principality is under our feet." Now the 'right hand' *is the place* of power and authority...the ruling and reigning of the Kingdom of the Great King!) As long as we believe this we will consciously or unconsciously accept the need to suffer. This is the old "pain is gain" doctrine.

But Jesus came to declare something very different. He said that the Kingdom or authority of the government of God, *the all good*, was deep within us already. He said that the Kingdom was here and now and already available simply by changing our minds, changing our thoughts, changing the direction we are looking. This is the process he called repentance. "Repent, for the Kingdom of Heaven is at hand." Repenting is the act of choosing a different way of thinking, behaving. It is not a protracted, convoluted emotion of unworthiness, as we have for so long been told. The simplicity of changing the direction of thought will cause us to enjoy the beauty, order and continual goodness of God with no fear of interruption... right here and now.

Why wait for something that we were intended to enjoy right now? Does our continual pain bring joy to God, our Creator? Does the suffering of your children bring you great joy? Is God served by our pain? Are we served by our pain? Only if we think we have something to gain by it. And that would be only if we don't believe that it is already here and now. "As in Heaven, so on Earth!" We foolishly look away from *now* to an experience far away and in the meantime allow the present pain to continue. If this were really true, why do we seek someone to make our pain go away? If we really believed we were to gain the glory of Heaven by our *purification through suffering,* why do we look for relief? Could it be because deep down inside we really don't believe that this is intended for us? Could it be because deep inside we carry the Spirit of Truth, the Mind of God and we really, on that level, know better?

It is true that "flesh and blood cannot enter the kingdom of heaven." We must be free of seeing ourselves as flesh and blood and begin to see ourselves as Jesus saw himself. One with the Father. Full of the Spirit of God. Created out from the Glory of God. Sent here to fulfill a Divine purpose. And all the while only as Beings of Eternal Light, Spirit beings! Then we would realize that we live in the Glory of the dominion of grace and Eternal Life.

Never accept a cause for suffering. Don't give it that validity. Mary Baker Eddy says, "It is nothing calling itself something." Just reject it from the start. Look away from it into the loving eyes of your Shepherd. Look to the allness of Divine Love. Look to that which cannot change nor be interrupted.

CHAPTER FIVE

WHAT IS HEALING REALLY?

"Out of your innermost being, rivers of waters flow.
Out of your innermost being, joy celestial flows.
Out of your innermost being, banishing all of your fears;
Out of your innermost being, Jesus the Christ appears."

"Whatsoever God has made shall be forever. Nothing can be added to it nor can anything be taken from it."
Ecclesiastes 3:14.

We must stop seeing healing as something being con-ferred upon us…something being added unto us that we don't have. We must stop seeing it as an illusive thing that we must obtain, find, get. This produces a very dangerous self serving (self-absorbed) and self grasping nature which springs from a thought that we are separated from our good and in need of trying to secure it….as opposed to the reality that we are already "complete in Him." As a matter of fact, we must stop seeing anything at all as something coming in from outside of us, something being added to us. Instead we must begin to feel what we need flowing *through* us.

When we read, "For *of* Him and *through* Him and *to* Him are all things," we get the image of an unbroken circle of grace and glory full of the abundance of all that is. And we are the *through* part. Out from His fullness and Majesty all things flow. We receive all things and give back to Him our love and devotion, gratitude and honor. Now realize that we are talking about this as something that is going on within our souls. God is the Life essence of us as well as of all Creation. This Life is within, without and fills all space. We live in it and it lives in us... and hopefully as we progress in our ability to yield to it...*as* us. This is how we experience the "oneness" that we hear so much about. It is not only a state of reality, but an experience as well. As a matter of fact, it is a necessary experience to healing.

We must begin to realize, to *feel*, that within us is all that pertains to Life, itself. We must instead begin to see wholeness, harmony and continual goodness as residing within us. "For of His fullness have we all received." "It is He who hath made us and not we ourselves"...and, "All the works of His hands are perfect." We contain all the attributes, characteristics, Wisdom, beauty and grace of God. This is the substance of our very being. We are not flesh and bones as we appear to be, but Light and Glory. We need to allow ourselves the *feeling* of being this Light and Glory. Let it rise from within us so that we may *feel* the wonders of its Presence within. Don't be afraid to do this, regardless of your present circumstances. This is the truth, *in spite* of your present circumstances.

≈

This Light and Glory must have free access of expression. Nothing must be allowed to obstruct its flow outward. When it is flowing freely, we are in health, in strength, in joy, in the experience of every good and blessed thing. We are happy, content, and living in the total absence of *needs*, or unfulfilled desires. When it is choked down or covered over, we are in darkness and misery, complacency, boredom, dis-ease. We feel separated from the good we need and we also feel personally responsible to fix whatever seems wrong.

If you will, take the time to read Chapter 47 in Ezekiel. It speaks of the flow of the Eternal Spirit of God as a fast, rushing river, flowing freely and *arising out from the depths of each soul.* You will realize that when this river of Eternal Life is flowing freely, everything in its path is touched and healed. There is no other "formula" for healing except to be in the flow of Life, itself. Every other "technique" is an admission of a lack of understanding and wisdom. It is palliative. It can only, at best, relieve present symptoms, yet leave the very consciousness which created the problem intact...only to resurface at a later time in perhaps another form. It is man trying to create Divinity. That is a pretty good definition of religion...man trying to reach or create Divinity. Instead of just *letting* Divinity express itself. And it will, it always will.

The flow does the healing. You don't and I don't. The essence of the Life which is flowing does the healing, the restoring, the rebuilding, the redeeming...and that will happen in a moment, in the twinkling of an eye, just as soon as the river is allowed free access.

ᴀ LEARN FROM
THE SEED

My yard at home is full of beautiful and majestic trees.
But the grandest of them all are the two black walnut trees
visible right outside my bathroom window. As autumn
progresses each year these trees drop hundreds of large, green
pods. Contained within these pods are the seeds themselves.
Black walnut seeds, to those who are not familiar, are the
hardest seeds to attempt to crack open. I have used a ham-
mer to do this in the past and usually unsuccessfully. We
drive over these pods with our cars and they remain intact.
But here is the wonder of it all.

As difficult as it surely is to open these from the outside, after they have remained in the earth for a season, they
crack open by themselves. And out emerges a tiny, white
sprout with its head humbly bent over. Now it is nonsense
for us to believe that this sprout cracked open the seed. One
could gently pinch a sprout and it would destroy it. A cat
could walk on a sprout and destroy it. In and of itself, the
sprout is impotent to even try. I like to think that this is
why it holds itself in such a humble fashion...to declare
that it has yielded to a power, an energy, a force greater
than itself. For deep within the seed is the Eternal Life of
every living thing. Deep within the seed is the same Life
that is deep within everything formed, including you and
me. It is the substance, the essence of the visible. There is
no strength in the visible. The power is in the invisible Life

within. When it is time for that Life to be revealed it will increase in intensity, expanding and magnifying itself until it implodes from within and begins to declare itself as a visible expression, in this case, the sprout. The sprout is but the visible expression of the Eternal Invisible. "For we have this treasure in earthen vessels, that the excellency of the power may be of God and not of ourselves." II Corinthians 4:7

With this same Power the way is *forged ahead* of the tiny sprout moving aside dirt and earthen clods in its path...thousands of times the molecular weight of the sprout. "I will send my Spirit before you and make the crooked places straight. I will break in pieces the gates of brass and cut in sunder the bars of iron." (Isaiah 45:2) We see this sprout appear through stone, boulders and even cement in its path. Nothing, no obstacle known to man, is able to stop its appearing...for the Life within and surrounding it is the Eternal Life of God.

If we focus on the pod or the seed, we lose. If we focus on the dirt, the heaviness, the obstructions to our good, we lose. If we focus on the millions of suggestions of the power of evil, we will lose. But if we focus on the Power, the Life, the Presence of the invisible God, we will always win!

Once my husband and I were visiting Alaska and had an occasion to view some of the magnificent mountains from a small helicopter. At one point on the tour we were taken over several dark, black granite-looking mountains where nothing grew. We were told that these were formed by the intense, hot lava from volcanoes which had erupted a very long time ago. Suddenly there appeared before us a mountain formed in the identical way, only this mountain was covered with soft, pale green grass. Our guide told us that this appeared only in the past few years. And I smiled and thought, "*I am* Life, and I will not be denied!"

No matter the appearance of evil, of long standing obstructions to goodness and abundance. No matter the name, the dreaded diagnosis, the list of thousands who have not been cured, the scientific brilliance that enshrouds the disease. If our focus is on the Life that never changes, that is uninterruptible and incorruptible, Eternal in the heavens...Life will certainly appear for us. Life will not be denied!

How is this uninterrupted flow of Life experienced?

I cannot speak of this without remembering the verse in Isaiah 25 which declares that there is a veil which is "cast over the faces of all nations" and as soon as that veil is removed, all disease, all sorrow, all sadness, all pain and human misery will cease to exit. Think of it! No human effort to correct or change anything at all. Only something obstructing which needs to be *removed...* and all we desire appears.

We, who have been raised in the age of scientific brilliance, are well versed in the belief that since disease is physical in appearance, it must be physical in origin and therefore, of necessity, physical in treatment.

But now, out from under the rubble of failed ideologies, comes the Eternal Knowledge that all disruptions to the experience of Love, life, harmony, goodness and order as coming from obstructions of thought and belief only. These evils now are evidences of internal obstructions, taught, believed and therefore experienced. And simple to remove.

Jesus was the first one to declare to us this truth when he said, "According to your faith (what you are believing) so shall it be done unto you." And, "As a man thinketh in his heart, so is he."

I think of Jesus at the tomb of Lazarus, when he instructed those who stood by to "remove the stone" which blocked the entrance to the tomb. And as soon as this was done, Life came forth with no struggle. Life with the full capacity to swallow up all appearances of death.

Another example of this concept is found in the study of Moses' "Tabernacle in the wilderness." The children of Israel knew nothing of possessing the Life and Glory of God. They knew nothing of being *one* with their Creator. And just as the religions of the world still project, they needed a place to go to worship their remote God. So God gave directions to Moses to build a tabernacle made of tents which could be carried along as they traveled about in their wilderness experience.

The whole thing was enormous in size. The majority of the space within this tent was called the "outer court" and most of the services conducted by the priests were done in this space.

The Israelites were allowed to roam this space freely. This speaks of the relationship that the far majority of people experience with God. However, contained within this large tent was a smaller tent comprised of two separate rooms. This was devoted to a much deeper service (or relationship) with God. Only few entered this room.

Within this first inner room were three pieces of furniture, each symbolizing a definite aspect of our experience with God, who is the Life of each one of us. One was called the Table of Shewbread, which speaks of eating (or partaking) of the hidden mysteries of God. "For unto you it is given to know the mysteries of the Kingdom of God." Only those who find a true desire towards God burning in their souls will enter this space in their hearts. The second is called the Candlestick, and it is a declaration that when we do partake of these hidden mysteries, our light is burning brightly, illuminating the souls of men and revealing the presence of the Kingdom of God (the reign of perfection and goodness.)

Finally the third piece of furniture is called the Table of Incense. It was positioned just in front of *the veil* which was the entrance into the last room, the deepest place of worship... The Holy of Holies. Incense is symbolic of the prayers and praises and deep devotion we offer to God as we enter His Presence. Within this veil, God dwelt.

Within the deepest recesses of the soul, the Spirit and Presence of God dwells. Within is the source and origin of our very existence. It is the place where Eternal, unending Life is realized. It is here we enter to obtain Wisdom and direction, clarity and understanding. It is here we find the wholeness we seek. It is here we find Life which knows no death. The children of Israel called this the Shekinah Glory of God. The radiance of this Glory was dazzling beyond description. The Glory was unspeakable.

The Presence filled this room and was contained within

by a veil of blue and gold, of magnificence and beauty. But the entire structure was covered by badger skin, a thick, grayish, mottled skin of no beauty at all. The symbolism is apparent. This skin, this covering, is symbolic of the human condition which covers and hides the Glory which resides within each of us. Only as this veil is split open can the Glory and the effects of it be realized upon the human condition.

Interestingly, this Shekinah Glory of God lived between two Cherubims seeming to guard it on both sides. It lived above another piece of furniture called the Arc of the Covenant. This contained, among other things, the Ten Commandments given to Moses by God, which is the law of sowing and reaping, sin equals death, cause and effect. The actual place and space of the residence of The Glory is called the Mercy Seat.

Again this is found above the Ten Commandments, saying to me and for all the world to know, that *Mercy excels over the law.* * * *That God deals with us in Mercy, *not according to our behavior,* but according to His never changing Nature of Mercy. Later in the New Testament we read "Mercy rejoices over judgment," and Jesus' words, "I will have mercy and not a life of sacrifices."

"The rain falls on the just and unjust alike." (The goodness of God falls on those who are living according to the Law of Love and those who are not.) This is Mercy! If there is any requirement at all for us to be able to receive the fullness of the goodness of God in our present circumstances, it would be that we are determined to be merciful to all people regardless of their present condition. We will cover this extensively later in the chapters on forgiveness and repentance.

So the upshot of all this is that we can know and expect goodness and Mercy, healing and the abundance of all good, *when this veil is removed*...not when we have earned anything, not when we have finally gotten it right, not when we finally say the right prayer, go to the right church, act in a certain way...or any other effort of man to reach or please God. It is all within and only needs to be allowed to express itself. To reveal itself. To flow.

The idea then is to remove something, not get something! In order to remove something we must follow the pattern set for us by Jesus who certainly removed all obstructions of the human condition for himself, as well as for us.

The "man born blind" from John, chapter 9, needed only to "wash away" the clay from his eyes and realize he was a spiritual being "sent" by God. (Speaking of the concept of mortality being replaced by the realization of perpetual immortality and Divine purpose.)

As this obstructing belief was washed away, he then began to see clearly who he was and why he was. His change came immediately as the veil of mortal identity was pierced and the radiance of immortality dawned. His "obstructing stone" was removed by revelation and by grace.

"For this mortal must put on immortality and this corruptible must put on incorruptibility." "Then it shall be said that 'death is swallowed up by Life.

༈ REMOVING
THE STONE

We need to look at how we block the flow. I call this the "open door" to allowing stuff we don't want to experience have access to our lives. But more important, we need to know how to fix this once it has happened.

One of the chief ways that we block it is not by what we do wrong so much as by what we are holding in our thought. Again, by what we are believing. Whatever we "put our faith in," is what we will experience.

People who come for help hope to be healed, but not all those really believe they will be. The task is to bring both hope and belief together and we do this by unveiling a new understanding, which when understood and adhered to will release the Life within and bring healing to any situation.

Here are some ideas commonly misbelieved.

We must stop seeing disease as a particular entity. It appears as something but really is nothing. It is really the *absence* of something. Just as darkness is the absence of light. Darkness is not a specific entity. It is the *absence* of something. I find it very helpful to see all disease as simply darkness.

I refuse to honor it with a name. Giving it a name and studying it with great detail only enshrines it. How badly do we want to be free of it? To that degree we will not grace it with a name, find a cause for it, or in any way elevate it in our mind. We must quickly *reduce it to darkness only*, before it gets an opportunity to create an image in our minds. Remember, "God has made man to walk 'upright' (as a prince, with power before God) but man has sought out many evil imaginations...or images."

All that appears as darkness or evil, is a *space* only, waiting to be filled with the Light and Glory of the Truth of the ever present, unchanging, Omnipresence of the Divine Life. I think of it as undeveloped land that has great potential and only needs cultivating. Remove all the undergrowth, trim the trees, plant new grass, spreading the seeds of truth and you have a picture of wholeness and beauty. Don't let your fearful imagination or the ignorant words of well meaning folks fill that "space." *You fill it*. You fill it with Truth and Love and every good thought. This is where the healing (or appearing of Life) takes place. You decide what will fill that space, not the doctor, lawyer, co-worker, spouse, friend or passer-by. You decide and that is exactly what will fill it.

A second common and deadly human belief.

We need to pause here and get something of great importance to be firmly established. God always wants Life to appear. God always wants to fill every space in consciousness with His Presence. God is infinite Life and Love and is ever expanding "from a boundless base." Wherever darkness is seen, Light is there to fill it. Love is there to fill it. God does not know a vacuum. You give Him that space to fill and He will fill it. But do not waver, wondering if God "has a good reason for this suffering." Do not dishonor God with such thoughts. *God never uses evil that good may appear.* Yes, it is true that when we turn to God with our whole heart good will appear where evil may have reared its ugly head. But God never was responsible for the evil to appear in the first place. God's will, God's intention, God's purpose is this: to *always* have Life and Love and Glory appear...regardless of the extent of the darkness, how long it has been in evidence, or what you may have believed in the past, or how much power you may have given to it in the past. Divine Love would have it no other way.

We must allow the Holy Spirit to sweep our souls and correct the myriads of false concepts we have held concerning the nature and intentions of Divine Love and Infinite Wisdom. Since time began man has distorted the very Image of the magnificence of God. We must make a deliberate intention to allow the Spirit to remove all that and replace it with what is Eternally true.

ॐ TRUE
HEALING

Healing then is simply allowing the Presence and the Power of the Spirit of God which resides within us, to flow out from us, making Itself manifested in the physical world.

As soon as we begin to see it this way it will be much easier for us to "have faith" or to believe that it will actually happen for us.

This is why.

The whole intention and purpose of God is to reveal LIFE to and through all physical forms. Remember that God is actually the Life force of every living thing. "For He is our life and the length (and strength) of our days." God is Life and Life is God. As God reveals the perfect Life, He is actually revealing Himself.

The Eternal Purpose and intention is to establish the Kingdom of God here on earth. What does that mean? It means to reveal the whole of Heaven right here in the physical world, "That God may be all in all." "As in heaven so in earth." We all have repeated those words thousands of times in our life every time we repeated the Lord's Prayer. Jesus taught us that this is the Father's intention. Always and in every situation…that Life would be revealed. All the beauty, all the radiance, all the Glory of Eternal Life, His life, to be made manifest. Remember that "Greater is the life that is within you than (anything that is in the realm of) that which is in the world."

Greater is the magnificence of the Glory of the Life of us all, than anything the world can hurl at us. Greater than any appearance of darkness… no matter how horrible it may be seen to be.

Dwelling in the confusion of "world thought," we will have "much tribulation." But we are instructed to "Be of good cheer, for I have already overcome it all!" And since the Spirit of Jesus is the Life of all that is and that Spirit resides within us and IS OUR LIFE…we can "be of good cheer" for He has already done what we are waiting to see happen. It is done. Nothing new needs to be done. It only must appear for us.

◈ THE ANSWER
TO IT ALL

One last human stumbling block is the scrambling, frantic, fretting efforts of man:

Now what is the driving force that makes it all appear? Grace. Not human effort at all. But only grace. "This mountain SHALL be removed, by my Spirit, says the Lord!" We are to "Cry, grace, grace unto the mountain and it shall be removed!"

"This mountain" being anything which stands before us to hurt or destroy, to deny that God is the ONLY power, and to blind us from the good that is available to us.

Now what is grace but the activity of the Spirit of God...the movement of the Spirit of God. It is the process by which the Life of the Eternal One is actually revealed to be the only power and swallows up the darkness that stands before us.

Grace is happening all the time throughout all of creation. But we don't see it until we yield to it. By that I mean until we start to trust it and acknowledge it.

We do this by stopping all human effort and "going with the flow" of grace. We stop resisting the evil. We stop fretting about it. We stop talking about it. We stop thinking about it. We will actually "feel" different. We will notice a definite shift in our thoughts and emotions when we have allowed grace to take over. We may be led to do something but it will not be an effort at all. It will feel so natural to us that we just "go with the flow."

Or we may *not* be led to do something, and that will cause us no concern. It will almost feel as though we don't care about the situation any more...but that, of course, is not true. It's just that we know it is taken care of and we do not need to be concerned again.

We will feel joy filling our hearts. It may seem strange

to feel joy in the midst of the confusion and darkness...but the truth is we won't see the darkness (as a power to hurt) anymore at all. We will be consumed by the grace and the Light of the Truth.

This is how healings happen. They happen from within our souls and burst forth into expression. *They always happen when all human effort has ceased.* And human effort ceases when we *choose to trust* grace.

Trusting grace is not as difficult as it sounds because now we are sure that the purpose of God is to come forth in this situation. Now we know for certain that the "will of God" is always LIFE. For God is the LIFE and it is this LIFE that fills all existence and gives everything expression.

A good exercise we can do is to choose to see Life everywhere. We learn to see not just trees, but the Life of the tree. We do this by a *feeling* more than a visual reality. We learn to see the Life of a child and not just the child running around. We choose to see the Life of the earth and not just a round ball of dirt and rock. We choose to see Life everywhere and in everything. Then it is not difficult to see the Life behind the disease, behind the darkness and destruction that is appearing.

Once we have developed the habit of seeing the Life of things instead of simply stopping with seeing the physical appearance, then it is easy to realize that the Life is always moving and active and pushing itself, if you will, into visible expression.

Our relationship with the earth and all that dwells upon it changes also. We begin to *feel ourselves* though life experiences, instead of charging through them. We have more respect for the holiness of the Life of others and less intolerance and judgment. We find ourselves feeling more respect for others and less criticism...because we begin to understand that we are dealing with God and not with a mortal man that seems to stand before us. We are dealing with God and not a sick, sinning mortal whose life has become a train wreck. This allows us to "call forth" the Son of God. To see it (with our heart) and to acknowledge its Presence and to encourage it to come forth...or to appear. This is what makes the healing happen. This is living by grace.

Now how do we get to this wonderful place in our souls? And why do we not trust grace immediately upon facing the dark and difficult challenges?

Probably the first reason we don't choose to trust is that we are not sure what we are supposed to be trusting. We have not developed a living relationship with our Creator and haven't had endless memories of continual victories during difficult times. Secondly, we have been taught and trained to think of God as the reason for our suffering. Even though we refute this, it is engrained into our hearts and raises its ugly head every chance it gets. Third, we don't fully understand the purpose and intention of God in human affairs. We don't fully realize that the whole scenario is for Life to be manifested through the darkness and established in the earth.

Right now I live in a home over looking a large lake. Actually we live immediately across from the enormous earthen dam which controls the water flow down the 'lower' Guadalupe River. I am amazed at the power of the water as it flows towards the dam. During one of the notorious floods we have here in Texas, the water rose over the 'spillway' to the right of the dam. It was the first time since the dam was built that the water reached spillway levels. Every few hours my husband and I would go out to the deck and watch the water as it roared over the land, taking with it every tree in its path. Finally there was only one large oak left and in spite of us rooting for it, it also yielded to the power of the river. Within three days the water had cut out a deep crevice in the earth which looked to all of us like a miniature Grand Canyon. During that flood 30 homes were swept away by the force of the water.Even now, whenever they open the gates to the dam, the water is released with such force that it arcs in the air over a city block long before it slams into the earth. The spray it creates reaches to the top of the trees.

I like to think of this scene when I remember the Power and Glory of God that lives within each one of us. I can visualize the intensity of the desire of God to release this Life-power and am fully persuaded that it only needs the slightest crack in the barriers we have inadvertently erected which block its flow. Once the way is cleared, even so minutely, the Light and Power is realized immediately and the visual appearance is corrected to reveal the perfection of all that God has formed. We call this a healing.

This is also called a healing by grace. Grace is, once again, the activity of the flow of the Spirit of God. What is created or revealed when the Spirit is allowed to freely express itself. The only real enemy to this free and easy flow of wonderment is "human effort." Every time we rush ahead to fix something, to talk about the power of the problem, to worry and fret...every time we use man-made ways and means to fix something, run to another mere mortal to fix us...or even use spiritual ways and means to "make something appear..." or to correct or change something, we are blocking grace from moving in our behalf. This is so critical to understand that before we talk about how to "remove the stone" we must address this.

"Should we ever use man's help?" Only if we are directed to do so. First, upon the realization of a problem, we must stop and remember. We must remember that God sent His Spirit to lead us and direct us to victory. We must remember that *our lives belong to God* and that Wisdom will be more than adequate to correct whatever has appeared.

So we stop and ask God for direction, for peace to be able to hear or feel the impulse of Spirit. At first this will be the scariest part of the whole situation. Maybe even scarier than the thing that threatens us. But this is only because we are challenging every distorted image about God that mankind has ever believed. We are standing before generations of mortal men who have spoken with authority things which are not true about God. We are refusing to be influenced by this again. We are choosing to put our lives before God and call Him Love! We are choosing to trust and believe even when we have not seen endless proofs of His uninterrupted Love for us. We stand and keep asking till the answer comes...and it always does. We mustn't think in our heart that we will not be able to hear the direction when it comes. God is Love and Love assumes responsibility to enable us to know. Just as a parent patiently teaches a child to understand words and direction, so much more does God. Isaiah chapters 30 and 31 deal extensively about this issue. As does a great portion of the Bible.

Most people that I deal with at the clinic have long ago come to the place where their trust and confidence in man's ways and means have vanished. But trusting in the leadership of God as their source of help is often still new to them. It is always my favorite part of helping them, to watch as this trust begins to unfold and flourish. These are the ones who are healed.

In Proverbs we read much about the value of leaning upon the Wisdom of God. It specifically declares that health, riches and honor, as well as long life is the reward for doing this. "Lean not unto thine own understanding, in all thy ways acknowledge Him and He shall bring it to pass." "Commit thy works unto the Lord and thy way shall be established." It is Wisdom to read the Book of Wisdom!

The footsteps to each healing will be by the activity of Spirit alone. We pause and ask, "What must I know here?" "What might be the obstructing stone in this particular situation?" It will not be the same as anything you have heard or understood before. In each situation the revelation, the answer, will be new and fresh. This is total surrender and total trust. We make space for the answer to appear and it always does. Again and again and forever.

CHAPTER SIX

GOING DEEPER INTO
THE LAW OF GRACE

The confidence we need to live in peace and the assurance of finding immediate help when we need it is found in understanding the Nature of the God who made us and who holds all of creation together. Why is this true? Because God deals with creation *according to His nature* and not according to how we live. This has confused mankind forever and is the cause of our not receiving all that we need freely and confidently.

We believe that we will receive the goodness of God only if we have earned it. We believe that if we don't "do right" or do everything perfectly or always stay centered and perfect in all our ways, we don't deserve blessings and help. Well, maybe we don't deserve it. But so what?! God deals with creation according to *His nature,* not according to our performance! This is hard to accept for some but let me try to explain it in a way that will help us all jump this necessary hurdle.

❦

In the Old Testament, before man was ready to understand His true and Eternal Nature... as a being created by Perfection and sustained by the Nature of Him who created us...mankind needed to be kept in order by an external law. And it was this law that was given to mankind through Moses. In the Wisdom of God, man needed this to keep him from inadvertently self destructing, and destroying one another. This law imposed external boundaries upon man and, as all law does, it contained rewards for keeping it and punishments for violating it.

Much like our traffic laws, let's say. If we keep the law, we find a certain degree of safety and a definite lack of punishment. If we break the law, we pay a fine or some other penalty imposed upon us. This will keep us from killing one another on the highways, and killing ourselves. Now hopefully the day comes in our maturing that we don't really need the law anymore because we have *become a law unto ourselves*. This means that I will drive my car in wisdom, in respectfulness towards others, and in sanity. I will do this because I have grown up and now it is *my nature* to want to drive this way. I don't do it any more because the law is present, but because it is now *my nature* to be mature and loving towards others on the road. I do it because it is "Wisdom" to do so.

The law of God is the same. We need it so long as we are still living out from a self destructive, selfish nature...which is the definition of the human consciousness or sin consciousness. But once we have tapped into a higher nature, which of course is our true nature, we "do right" because it is our nature to do so.

So we read in the book of God's Wisdom, in Galatians, that man lived under the law "until Christ was come." At which time he no longer needed the law because he now had become a law unto himself. The phrase, "until Christ is come," is referring to the time when we, each one, individually and collectively, come to the place where we realize that our nature is the Wisdom and Love of God and no longer lawlessness and ignorance. Christ truly comes, or appears, as we accept our Oneness with him and in him.

This is why Jesus came... to bring to mankind the realization of his (man's) true nature... as lived by the Power of the Holy Spirit only. So again we read, "The law came by Moses, but grace and truth came by Jesus Christ." Jesus ushered in a whole new way of living. Living by Love. Living by the Nature of the God who has chosen to "tabernacle in man." And the power to do this is found in the flow of the Spirit of God *and no other.*

So "John (the Baptist) came to baptize you with water unto the remission of sin, but there is one who has come who will baptize you with the Holy Spirit and with fire (passion)." A whole new era for mankind was born with those words.

No longer does man need to fear punishment or to fear that the help he needs will be withheld from him. God deals with us, not according to our righteousness, but according to His righteousness. As a matter of fact, we read these startling words, "We are the righteousness of God in Christ!" so if God sees us through the lens of His own pure Nature, then why would there be a need for punishment?

It is God's Nature to love. It is Love's nature to give. It is Love's nature to show Mercy. As a matter of fact, Mercy is His name! And Mercy is the ability to look beyond the appearance or the picture and to deal according to the Eternal nature (and not according to 'earning.')

My favorite analogy is the sun. "The sun shines on the just and the unjust," we read in Luke. And "The rain falls on the good and on the evil alike." This is the definition of Mercy and how God deals with us. God is like the sun that shines on the most generous deed as well as the most heinous deed alike. The Psalmist says that the Mercy of God is from ever lasting to ever lasting. God always pours out goodness for it is His Nature to do so. He cannot do anything contrary to His Nature. Now, whether we receive this, or can even *accept* perpetual goodness, is entirely dependent upon us (by grace). If we choose to live in the shade, we can't complain that the sun isn't shining. If we stay indoors, we may not feel it or benefit from it, but it is always shining for us just the same.

So how do we gain from this perpetual goodness? One, we recognize that it exists for us. We recognize that we don't have to earn it, nor indeed *can we* earn it at all. As a matter of fact, if we insist upon trying to earn it, we will be "putting ourselves back under the law." There is no Mercy in the law! Second, we prove that our nature is His Nature by showing Mercy to others. Even the most depraved. Even the ones who have hurt us the most. This enables us to be "open" to receive the Mercy we need.

Here is another favorite analogy…do we tip at a restaurant because the wait person deserved it or because it is our nature to give from our heart? Are we treating others according to their "earning" in our sight, or out from our merciful nature? If we tip according to how they have earned it in our sight, we are insisting that they *earn* our gift. If we insist that another earns his gift, then we have put ourselves under the same law and we cannot receive from God freely and immediately. We will unconsciously be judging ourselves in the same way we have judged another. We also will feel the need to "earn" our goodness. We will be standing in the shade wishing we could feel the sun, wondering what it will take for God to give to us.

We might even be very foolish and find ourselves trying the hundreds of human ways and means to "make a healing happen." This is living "under the works of your own hands." And it is futile. Hebrews, chapter 3 and 4 spends a lot of time explaining this to us.

"He who has *ceased from his own works* (trusting God to be the goodness they needed) has entered into the 'rest' of God." This means that he who yet lives by his own works will "die in the wilderness" as the Israelites did so long ago, for they did not understanding the Nature of God, (therefore they did not understanding their own nature, made in His image.) Not knowing the goodness and Mercy of God, they trusted in their own efforts to live. It is in the 'rest' of God (state of absolute trust) that healing becomes spontaneous. Trust comes by knowing that God pours out from the abundance of His goodness, notwithstanding any effort on our part to achieve it.

❧

The proof that you have accepted that God is always merciful is that under all conditions you will be merciful to others. You choose to give to those standing on the corner begging "as unto the Lord." You silence the judgment that says, "They could get a job just like me." You see Jesus standing there instead of the man and you choose to show Mercy. For you see, neither have you measured up to the Nature of God in your life and you want Mercy, right? So you show it to others, as well.

The ability to do this does not come from man. It comes as a result of the Presence of the Holy Spirit which lives within you and is the very Life of God within you. As you choose to live this way, the Spirit enables you to live this way. We choose, He appears! We desire to live out from our true nature and He fulfills that desire. This is grace. There is no other way.

CHAPTER SEVEN

OMNIPOTENCE AND WORSHIPPING STRANGE GODS

Are we striking out right and left trying to make something go away? Or trying to change something? Are we fearing or fretting? Have we tried every imaginable and unimaginable human ways and means and the problem persists?

Our problem is that we first believe that the problem is a real power, able to hurt us. We see this thing standing before us as a viable threat to our well-being...or the well-being of someone else. If we didn't see this as a real threat, why would we be trying to make it go away? Why wouldn't we just move on with our lives and let it be?

Once again we read, "Whatsoever we fear, that also we worship." To whatever we attribute power, to that we believe ourselves subservient. It then has begun to rule our lives... to destroy if it chooses. We put ourselves under the authority of whatever we believe is a power that can rule our affairs. This could be a "thing" or a person, a condition or an event.

Once we come to a measure of understanding of what is true and what is false, we may try to *use that truth* against the problem. Are we using these truth principles as weapons to defeat the appearance of evil? If we are doing this we are giving the evil appearance power to rule over us. Unless we thought it was a valid power to hurt us, why would we be throwing the words of truth against it?

All this is worshipping "strange gods." Defined as giving a fearful moment to a disease, a person, a circumstance or an event we imagine can hurt us.

There is only One God and only One Power. This Power is all about goodness, harmony, balance, order and abundance. It has one objective, one goal...and that is to establish in the visible world what is already present in the world of the Eternal invisible.

Actually it knows only this Present Perfection as already being in a state of perpetual, uninterruptible, incorruptible order and magnificence. It is *we* who are looking out at darkness and trying to chase it away. But since God is the only Life, the only Power, the only Mind, the only manifestation, the only Creator...since God is "above all, in all and through all" and we are living and moving and having our existence within this Allness...we cannot be separated from the Mind which only knows perpetual Light and Glory, goodness and joy. It is our mind. We don't have two minds...one for truth and one for confusion. We have only the Mind of God who already knows and is at perfect rest with its present perfection. "For you have the mind of Christ."

So where do these gross, darkened thoughts which grab

our imaginations and become for us appearances of horror, actually come from? They come from spaces in consciousness which have yet to be filled with what is true and real. "And the Earth (referring to mortal thinking) was without form and *void* and darkness covered the face of the deep." This is talking about our state of awareness...what we perceive as real...otherwise known as "consciousness."

"And the Lord said, 'Let there be light.'" When the truth is apparent the light of that truth shines on the darkness and confusion... and it vanishes. So we read, "The truth shall make you free."

Jesus said he was that Light. He certainly brought awareness and clarity to the human, darkened understanding. He introduced the true Nature of God and the true nature of man to be one. He showed that the "Kingdom," or ruling authority, was already present for perpetual good. ("The Kingdom of God is here, now, and is within you all." And, "Of His fullness have we all received." He also said that as we were consciously one "in Him" we were that Light as well...sent to shine upon every appearance of darkness to prove the Omnipotence of God. To be "in Him" is to be One with the Mind, the understanding, the knowing that he possesses...which is the Eternal Mind of God. As we draw upon this understanding, we are manifestations of that Light. "He is the Father of Lights with whom is no variableness (changeableness) nor shadow of turning." And, "He is the true Light which lights every man who comes into the world."

The horrific things we perceive, that which we experience or see all around us, is a result of living out from an unenlightened, darkened understanding. This is why it is said that Jesus came to destroy the "sin" consciousness...which is the darkened understanding.

Again we read in Ecclesiastes that "God made man to 'walk upright'"... or to rule in the authority of God... but that "man has sought out many evil imaginations." So here we understand that the evil we see comes from the imagination or "imaging" of a mind ruled by confusion, devoid of light.

Thus we are told to "Bring every thought into captivity to the mind of Christ." "In your patience possess ye your souls." Every time we face a destroying thought...knowing that there is only One power and that is the power of good...we shine the Light of Heaven, the truth of Eternal, perpetual goodness, upon that space in consciousness. From that moment that space is forever secure in the Light, as the Light. It could be likened to a house with many doors. Every time a door is opened that has not been opened before we face darkness. It might appear as a relationship gone haywire, a disease process, a financial impoverishment, a terrific weather event, an accident, or whatever...*how it appears is not the issue anymore*. It was an issue as long as we thought these things were real and could actually hurt us! But now we treat these things as thoughts, imaginations, just darkness. So how it appears is not to be the issue. Now there is only one issue. We shine the light by asking, Where is the power?

The only Power, the absolute only influence, is God, the Eternal goodness. No matter what or how evil appears, there is *one factor in the equation only*....where is the power here? As we stand facing the evil and know we are the Light of the truth of the One Power of God...we shine that Light upon the evil and the evil vanishes. But if we flail and flurry, worry or fret, race and run for someone to do something...no matter what comes out of our mouth...our actions show we yet believe in other gods, strange and aberrant, obtrusive and powerful....and we as their victims!

As we stand worshipping and adoring the One and Only influence over and through His creation...we find peace melting over us, confidence and assurance rising up from within us. We don't need to utter a sound. Life is God and God is our Life. Therefore, nothing, absolutely nothing can interrupt the steady flow of this One Life. Lots of things will threaten to be able to do so. But as we stand remembering our life is "hid in Christ in God..." "It is he who has made us and not we ourselves" And, "When Christ shall appear, *Who is our life...*"

When we remember we posses no life of our own but all is a manifestation of the One Life and that is the "fullness of God"...then the Light shines into the darkness "and the darkness cannot grasp it" (overcome it.)

Are we lifting our thought, straightening our back, squaring our shoulders and being the object of Love's care? Are we honoring the only reality that is possible?

Our decision will master us, whichever direction it takes.

Will we allow this circumstance, event, person, to have even one moment of mastery over us? Are we allowing it to own our souls? Will this symptom, this name (of apparent affliction) have ownership over our bodies? Who owns the body? Who owns the soul?

Are we pawns to the circumstance? Or are we the ever present, ever active, Holy Sons of God sent here to dispel all darkness by the radiance of the Light that we are? Are we the visible expressions of the invisible, uninterrupted Eternal Life?

Even in the darkest times the fact is *One Life alone governs the moment.*

Is this to be an experience of death or despair to us? Or are we created to experience the power of the resurrected Christ in our awareness or consciousness?

If you feel instructed to do something, say something, go somewhere, etc...that will come later...only after the Omnipotence of the Omnipresence of the One Life has been firmly established in your soul.

Recently a lovely woman who is currently a patient at the clinic made this profound statement, one I will never forget. Initially diagnosed with an incurable illness and given only months to live, she has defied these predictions by this realization, "My change came when I realized that I had a choice!"

Amen!

Chapter Eight

REPENTANCE, FORGIVENESS AND REALIZING YOUR ETERNAL PURPOSE

The Spirit of God flows throughout Eternity as a mighty river of beauty and strength. Even when the current seems to slow down, beneath the surface the river runs strong. You cannot see this river, but just like the wind which also cannot be seen, you will always feel the effects of its Presence. When you can feel this uninterrupted Presence you will then realize wholeness, strength and completeness. The secret is in the realization of it, for it is always present. It is the *Life of all things and by it all things consist*...are held together. It is the Life of you and me and everything created, seen or unseen.

When we find ourselves overcome by a situation, that sense of being overcome is a clear indication that we are not realizing the Presence of this Spirit of Life. We will face many adverse circumstances as we travel through this period, but we were never supposed to be overcome by them. When we take our attention off the Spirit of Life and look fearfully at the threat, we are overcome. When we look once again towards the Light of Glory, which is our very Life, we are victorious. Really it is that simple.

Many things will temporarily block the flow of this Life through us, but none so completely as an unforgiving spirit. There is a reason that this is true. But first, the definition of forgiveness is "to send away." Not just to send away the offense, but also the repercussions from the offense. One sincere act of forgiveness washes the whole mess clean, just as if it never happened. A sincere act of forgiveness is the purest expression of Love we will ever experience or give. It has the capacity to heal the worst of human conditions. I have seen multitudes of instant healings throughout my lifetime by this simple act of forgiveness. This is true Mercy, to choose to "send away" both the sin and the judgment due. Until someone does this for us, or we do it for ourselves or others, we will reap what we have sown, whether we have offended deliberately or ignorantly. It is in forgiving, sending this away, that we find ourselves able to go forward without repeating the offense again and again. The sense of condemnation, guilt, and fearful looking for the punishment...all strengthens the offense. The *removal* of it all frees us to live above it.

* *Forgiveness is the tool used to heal disease appearances as well as offenses committed.* We are taught to have pity on those who suffer from disease...and rightly so. But we stop there, believing we are impotent to help them. We must realize that behind the appearance of disease is the belief that there is a power of evil that can usurp the Presence and authority of God. We must know that this is dishonoring God and is the root of all disease. It is idolatry to

give such power to evil. It is exalting disease...it is in a sense worshipping it...even though we hate it. Revelations declares that "Whatsoever you fear, that also you worship." Therefore, we forgive the suffering soul--or release the belief in the pre.... of evil-- and both the belief and the repercussions of that belief (sickness) is removed.

We speak of disease with such reverence. We build huge edifices to each specific appearance. We spend billions of dollars, often our entire savings in response to its lies of power and magnitude. We think about it day and night. We talk about it day and night. It consumes our lives, whether we are experiencing it or not. This is rank idolatry! And this must be repented of. This is where we should start with every healing we desire. To repent of spending our entire lives, or even one moment, giving power to such darkness and confusion. Know that this simple act of repentance will wipe the years of such belief away in an instant and *make room* for God in all the Glory of Eternal Power and Perfection to appear. "Nothing can enter in (to the Kingdom of God) that believes or makes a lie!" We need to repent of it and then deliberately send it away from us, from our experience, from our lives! This is the full circle of repentance and forgiveness.

We must not withhold forgiveness, simply because in doing so we halt the flow of Life through our very own souls. The minute we choose unforgiveness we choose for our own death!

Not everyone feels comfortable forgiving another. Some choose to wait till the offending person has suffered enough to satisfy his/her idea of justice. To those who are loath to allow someone to "get away with sin without punishment," they will also find themselves receiving punishment with no Mercy when they need it the most. For who has not needed Mercy in their lives?

But to those who love Mercy... and realize that "Mercy rejoiceth against judgment,"... they will live in the Mercy of God.

Jesus said to the religious leaders of his day, "I will have Mercy and not a life of religious sacrifice...go and learn what that means!"

Micah, the prophet, announces this word from the heart of God, "I will show thee, Oh man, what is good and what does the Lord require of thee, but to do justly and to *love Mercy* and to walk humbly with thy God."

Time and time again, page after page, we are instructed to show Mercy and not be swift to punish. Punishment may stop the immediate problem, *but it can in no way correct the consciousness that was present to commit the offense.* Change and correction comes by Mercy and not by exacting judgment.

A word of wisdom and caution...while the desire to show Mercy may live in your heart, the time to demonstrate it is from the Lord. Meaning, we must wait till we know when the perfect timing is apparent before we rush to show the Mercy we feel. The heart and soul of the offender must have been made ready to receive this or he will take this as an occasion to continue offending. In cases such as this, hold your peace till the time is right and you will surely know it. Never are we to be led by human emotions in this work, but only as the Spirit leads us. When the ground is made ready by the Spirit of God, the time will be right to plant the seed of Mercy. To do this prematurely is foolish and defeats the purpose, which is to heal and restore the soul of the offender.

The "battered woman" is a classic example of forgiving prematurely for the sake of immediate peace. This is not being led by the Wisdom of God but by a foolish desire to live in peace at all costs. This is also seen in world affairs. To forgive an offense prematurely, before the recipient is repentant, is to invite further disasters. And only God knows the hearts of men. So we wait on him, not desiring punishment, but not running from it either...always waiting for the opportunity to forgive.

ॐ UNDERSTANDING OUR DIVINE PURPOSE

To fully understand the importance of forgiveness we must examine why we are here. We must know the Eternal purpose and infinite intention of God who sent us here for His purposes. Otherwise all this will only be an exercise in religion.

Who are we? Why are we here? What is God's intention for our existence on this mortal realm?

When asked by the religious leaders of his day how He was able to perform such miracles, Jesus answered, "You know not who you are, where you have come from or why you are here." Meaning, with this knowledge we also would be equipped to heal others.

Who are we?

We are all created out from the midst of the realm of God. This is our source, no matter our human story. We are demonstrations, manifestations, declarations and definitions of the Life which spawned us. As we embrace this truth we reflect this Life, all its characteristics and attributes, all its Wisdom and might. Deep inside we realize this, which is why we long to contact this realm again throughout our lives. It is a desire to return to our home so to speak. Our place in Spirit where we are BEING who we are. It is this reality which causes us to know that there "must be more than this." It is this reality which, when understood and embraced, even if we don't "feel it" yet, that allows us to heal others. This is what gives our word power. This is what gives authority to our intentions. Without the realization of our true identity, we will forever feel "outside" of God and in need of His favor, in need of Him "fixing us." But with this realization we feel One with God and One with His wholeness and fullness, never feeling separate from all that He is. Never needing to be "fixed," we live out from the uninterrupted expectation of perpetual goodness.

Why are we here?

We are sent here as the Eternal Light of God to bring this Light to any and all darkness that appears in our path...that God may fill all space with His power and Presence. In the first chapter of Genesis we read that "The earth was without form and void and darkness covered the face of the deep." This is referring to the human condition we are sent to. The mass consciousness that covers the earth like a blanket of darkness, chaos, and deep confusion. In this state of darkness every evil imagination is declared to be reality. The truth, the Light, is not seen so whatever is imagined is believed.

The solution is the appearing of the Light of the absolute truth that God is good and goodness rules its creation in order, harmony and present perfection. That God is Omnipotent...the all and only power. That mankind can expect goodness and live out from it forever. That, in Joel Goldsmith's words, "Man was not born to cry."

We have been sent to *deliver this truth*, to *prove this truth*, to restore mankind to its "right Mind" relieving it from its present state of fearful insanity. This is our job. This is God's purpose for our Being. "I have created you out from my image. Go now and take dominion over the earth. Subdue it. Bring it to peace and harmony. I have given you authority over all the works of darkness. You are the Light of the world. In your mouth is the power to restore, rebuild, and redeem mankind. Be who you are!" We fulfill this by forgiveness. Seeing beyond the disease/offense unto the ever present Son of God is one demonstration of forgiveness. Releasing and "sending away" the invading thought, suggestion, and evidence of evil is the second form that forgiveness takes.

There are many these days who announce that our greatest purpose and achievement is to serve ourselves, to gain as much for ourselves as we can. And we do this by using the sacred and Eternal Principles of Truth. This also is rank idolatry. "Take no thought for your life...for your Father knows what you have need of. But seek first the Kingdom of God and His righteousness, His Divine Purpose, (all he has purposed for your being) and all this will be added unto you." Seek first to fulfill your Divine Purpose, to heal, to show Mercy, to serve God daily..."For those who would seek to gain in this life, will lose... and those who seek to put the purposes of God first in this life, will gain."

The means of fulfilling this holy purpose is forgiveness. By the deliberate act of "sending away" the darkness and declaring a person's rightful inheritance, all confusion, all evil, all pain, all misery is cancelled and the person is able to awaken into his/her right Mind. As we choose to deny whatever appearance is declaring itself a power and see the person as Love Itself, Life Itself...we are fulfilling the purpose for which this has come into our path! We can only do this as we deny any desire for revenge or "just punishment."

Isaiah 61 begins with this statement of truth. "The Spirit of the Lord is upon me. He has anointed me to preach good tidings to the meek. He has sent me to bind up the broken-hearted, to proclaim liberty to the captives, and the opening of the prison to them who are bound."

Jesus said, "As my Father sent me, so send I you. Heal the sick, raise the dead and cast out demons...free my people!"

This is why Mercy is so critical. It is the act of removing the offense (forgiveness) without the intention or desire to inflict punishment or pain. It is the "Goodness of God that leads men to repentance." Not the pain they are presently experiencing.

As we take on the heart of Mercy, we find the ability to heal rather simple. We choose to see beyond their offense, beyond their belief in the power of disease, beyond their fears and beyond whatever is manifesting because of their beliefs and fears...right through it all! We choose to see *in them* that which never changes...indeed cannot change or be altered in any way...for the true substance of their Being is the Light and Glory of God. "Whatsoever God has made shall be forever. Nothing can be added to it, nor can anything be taken from it."

This is true forgiveness. It may start as a superficial act of letting go an offense, but must finally reach the pinnacle of reality for the healing to appear.

What blocks us from doing this?

Mostly ignorance. We find ourselves lost in the same mind of insanity that we were sent to remove. We find ourselves groping in the same darkness and confusion we came to relieve. We find we also are dazzled by the appearances of evil and we, too, are embracing it all as a power *other than God*. Until the "Word of the Lord comes" and we are awakened out from our long sleep and begin to realize who we are and why we are. Until we feel the stirring of the Spirit of Light and Glory, the Spirit of Wisdom and dominion. Then only can we shake off the grave clothes and step up to the plate.

The best description of the condition of the world thought is the "victim mentality." The world is lost in its imaged victim-hood. Afraid of disease, destruction, accidents, and death...everything becomes a potential enemy to be dreaded, feared. The seasonal changes, the trees, the grasses, the pollen, the microorganisms...afraid of the very earth which was created to sustain us. The victim mentality knows no bounds in its paranoid insanity. It is afraid of everything and everyone who walks and breathes. It is especially afraid of the body given to us, to serve us here, during this present time. Have you ever watched a bird sitting at a feeder? Its little head is jerking here and there, nervous and fearful, watching for the sudden appearance of larger birds. This reminds me of the condition of those who have yet to realize the indescribable wonders of who they are and the Glory of the earth with which we share our lives.

❧ FORGIVENESS BEGINS WITH REPENTANCE

"For why do you seek to remove the mote in your brother's eye and leave the beam in your own? First clear the beam out from your own eye and then you can see clearly to remove the mote from your brother's eye."

We cannot help anyone if we are yet lost in the same consciousness they are. If we also feel fear, if we also feel anger and resentment, if we also stand in shock and horror at appearances of evil, we cannot deliver others. When we can look at the evil appearance and know that it is simply a thought, a belief, and not a power at all, then we are equipped to help.

How do we get there? What if we have held past resentments? What if we also cringe at the name or manifestation of disease? What if we are seeing evil as a power, just as the one coming to us for help?

First we must deal with our own sin. And sin it is... to

give power to anything other than God, Good. If we are re-acting at all, we need to clear our own soul first. The simplicity of getting out from under this effect is repentance.

To pause for one moment and pray, realizing and confessing that we are *seeing this evil as a power greater than God*, to accept that there even is a power *other than God*, to acknowledge that we are experiencing fear or anger (same thing)...and then to "send it away from our soul" is the first step to any healing. One moment of clear thinking, one moment of sending it away...demanding it leave...will be all it takes. It will leave! It may try to come back, especially if you have held the belief for a long time, but just keep repeating the prayer, sending it away and finally it will go and stay gone.

One of my favorite stories to illustrate this principle is about a lady who prayed, and sought out others to pray, for her husband who was a severe alcoholic for 40 years. The children had come and gone only knowing their father as an alcoholic. Now the grandchildren were being raised with the same influence. The wife continued to be desperate. Finally one day, after literally years of begging, he agreed to go to an AA meeting. She was ecstatic and happily went with him. After the meeting was over many of the folks who often attended gathered around this new couple to welcome them and to encourage them to return. Suddenly it occurred to the wife that they might think that she was the one with the problem. So to make sure they knew it was him and not her, she said, "I have been asking him to come to one of these meetings for 40 years now!" There was a moment of silence as the others took in the obvious reason that she said this. Remember that these folks have been around the block several times concerning this in their lives and not much will get past them. Finally a woman put her hand on the wife's shoulder and said, "My, but we are a martyr, aren't we!" The wife was incensed, humiliated and caught!

That night she stayed awake and reflected on what actually happened there. She had to admit that she was seeking not to be labeled as the alcoholic, for such a label and life-style was disgusting to her. She began to pray and ask God to reveal to her what she needed to know here. Her answer was immediate. She needed to repent for the judgment and condemnation she held for her husband. Her condescending attitude was clearly blocking her from seeing the real man...and healing him. She was filled with remorse and truly realized what she had fallen into. She determined to pray steadily for four months (the whole summer) not for her husband, but for herself. She realized she needed to remove the mote in her own eye! And faithfully she did just that.

Well into the four months her husband noticed a definite change in her attitude towards him. She began to remember the wonderful qualities she saw in him when they first married. She began to appreciate the overwhelming goodness of his nature and her heart softened towards him. She never mentioned the drinking again.

I'm sure you have guessed the outcome here. He began to respond to her love for him and his heart began to change as well. He stopped drinking after 40 years, never drank again.

When we are able to see beyond the disease, the offense, the sin...and realize the wonders of the man created in God's image and heart, that will be what appears. It is a principle that never fails!

Conversely if we are still seeing the disease, the offense, as a power to overcome, we must realize we are blocking the healing for the person (or ourselves) and we must begin by acknowledging that we are denying God as the all and only Presence and Power...and then release that thought from our soul. Otherwise the grace, the flow of strength and love and power cannot flow, and healing cannot appear.

ᔥ MAKING SPACE

With the way cleared, with the soul unburdened and now free, you have "made space" for God to occupy. Two opposing thoughts cannot occupy the same space at the same time. We cannot be living in the realm of evil vs. good and the absolute state of the fullness of Divine Life at the same time. When one is gone the other will surface immediately. The fullness of God is within you. It only waits for space to surface and occupy. Providing that space by repentance it will suddenly fill your heart and mind with faith and confidence. You are then ready to heal, to forgive, to be who you are.

This is the tool Jesus spoke of when he said that the way into the Kingdom of power and peace is repentance. The Kingdom or rule of authority and power is within us.

We are in it as well. "In him we live and move and have our being." This Spirit and Presence is all around and about us. It flows through us. We realize and "feel" it doing so when we "make space" for it to appear. The effect of one sincere moment of humility and repentance will immediately provide that space.

Too often people start right in trying to heal something by speaking the truth, demanding it appear, over and over again affirming what they know and believe is the absolute truth. But they yet fail. If this is the case, the reason is they did not take time to clear the space for grace to appear. The works are done by grace and grace alone. *It is the activity of the Spirit of God on the human condition.* Grace will do whatever needs to be done. But for grace to appear, we must make the space available. Human effort, struggling and squirming, will never accomplish what we desire. Only the soft and sure, confident and quiet Presence of grace. This is how grace is activated.

Again, "It's not by power (human), not by might, but by my Spirit. And you shall cry 'grace, grace' unto this mountain which stands before you. And this mountain *shall be* removed, by my Spirit, saith the Lord."

Step one then is to make space available by the removal of suggestions of evil as a power. But step two is to deliberately allow and visualize the space you have provided, now filled with the abundance, the wholeness and the fullness of God.

You can readily see that the majority of the work is done in the quiet and silence of our own soul. The evidence of healing is simple once the ground has been prepared for the seed of the Spirit and Word of truth. Always the ground must be made ready before the seed can be sown. This is the effort, the preparation of the heart, not the actual healing at all. The seed grows without the effort of man. Our job is in the preparation of the soil.

We must forgive all and everyone. We must bless them with a true and honest blessing from the heart of God. We must honestly want them to be made whole. As we do this we clear our own souls as well. We are fulfilling God's purpose and intention for our appearing, at this moment, in this place.

CHAPTER NINE

MAKING THE SEPARATION

When dealing with any diseased condition, let's look at what is really going on here. I call this belief "learned insanity" and this is why.

We know that we are formed and created by Eternal Perfection. "It is He who has made us and not we ourselves." We know that "all the works of His hands are perfect." We know that we are a manifestation of the Eternal, uninterrupted, incorruptible, radiant Life that is God. We are made of the same stuff, the same substance, attributes, nature and total characteristics of God. "Of His fullness have we all received."

Once again we read in Ecclesiastes, "Whatsoever God has made shall be forever. Nothing can be added to it nor can anything be taken from it."

Now if all this is true, and it is, then how could disease or any confusion in appearance, or mind, exist? The answer is of course, "It can't!"

So all darkness and confusion, disease and disruption

must be something other than what is seen. Since there is only One Power, One Divine Influence, all disease and other manifestations of evil are only "suggestions" of another power. These suggestions are thoughts, fears, and images of horror which we have learned (and therefore believed) were real.

In the beginning of this visible world, God defined the "thought" or level of consciousness we were to be sent to. He called it "without form, void, and chaos and darkness covered it." We were sent to be the Light unto this darkness. To be the Order to the confusion. To be the living Truth, a testament to the Power of only God, goodness. We call this space the human consciousness. The Bible calls it the sin consciousness. Sin here meaning the consciousness of being a separate entity from all that God is... from God Himself. We are sent here to fill this voided space with Light, with truth.

To the degree that we are able to remain poised in the face of the darkness, however it may appear...to that degree will we bring light and the darkness will flee. But if and when we "hear" the suggestion of a power, of a condition, of a disease and believe the physical evidence, believe the suggestion of power...to that degree we become enslaved by the appearance, by the belief. The minute we give it a name, give a reason to exist, we have become enslaved.

But to those who are wise, it remains *outside* of them...only a suggestion. They may *see* it... in or on their bodies. They may *feel* the effects of it. But all this seeing and feeling is only *coming from the suggestion itself*...definitely not from *within* the holy, uninterrupted life of the Son of God.

So when we seek a healing, we are declaring that we have already "bought into" the lie. First we have believed it is real. Then we have believed that it can interrupt the very image and expression of God. And then we have forgotten totally who we are and why we have come and we become, in our minds, victims of this madness.

This is why Jesus said in Matthew 25 that we should visit him when "in prison." The prison being *the belief of enslavement to darkness.*

In the Bible these suggestions of evil are called "evil spirits." By naming it so mankind could more easily realize that they were dealing with an external suggestion and not a real condition. They could then still see themselves as intact, whole and impregnable to hurt. They could see this offending evil as *outside of them* and not a part of them at all. The next step is easy then. It simply becomes a matter of sending it away...along with every appearance, every feeling, and every thought. Now it is seen to be only an external suggestion and therefore easy to send away. Remember that "sending away" is the true definition of "forgiveness." We forgive ourselves, we forgive others, every time we realize the bad behavior, the diseased condition, etc., is not coming from them or us, but is some annoying suggestion that can be sent away.

The real truth is that harmony never needs to be restored, for it is forever intact. But the belief in an interruption of harmony needs to be removed. We don't need something fixed, but we do need it removed.

When my second daughter was still an infant and toddler, among all her other problems she was severely cross-eyed. Especially in one eye which I was later told was blind. Every time I looked at her and her eye was crossed I would say, "Honey, don't do that." In her infant state she, of course, would have had no idea what I was referring to and I never said. But I was consistent...and that is a key factor. Every single time that eye would cross I said it. I was telling her she had the ability not to allow that manifestation of confusion. Strangely enough, every time I said it, she would blink and straighten out her eye. Finally she just quit being cross-eyed at all. What I didn't realize till later, the eye began to see as well. When she had trouble breathing, I told the external influence of evil to just leave her alone. It always left right away, as did fevers, and all other manifestations of confusion. Sometimes they stayed away forever. Sometimes they came back and I needed to say it again. But I always experienced complete victory.

I have before told the story of Toni, but it seems appropriate to repeat it here. She is a middle aged women who had a urinary bladder "condition" (suggestion) called interstitial cystitis. The names are always an attempt to exalt the condition and validate its existence. Anyway, she suffered pain, burning and frequency of urination day and night for 11 years with no let up. The medical suggestion was to remove the bladder and have her wear bags on the side of her body to collect the urine, so she, like so many before her, refused. One night at a meeting we were having she really grasped this concept of being separate from the condition...that it was really a suggestion and not a condition within her at all. During that night she awakened to the typical pain and this time she played the game, "Knock-knock" with the suggestion. She said, "Knock-knock. Who's there?" The reply was "pain." She said, "What do you want?" and the answer came, "To make your life miserable." So she told it that it was not welcome, that it was an intruder into her home and that it needed to leave. The next thing she heard was, "Why? You have always let me in before?" To which she firmly replied, "Never again!"

She told us she needed to repeat this a total of four times that night, every time it tried to return. She never felt it again for four months! It tried to return once then, she repeated the same thing, and this time it never returned. After 11 years, with only the understanding that this condition was not a part of her, not what it seemed to be, but actually an external intruder, she was able to easily separate herself from it altogether.

Recently we began working with a very young child who was having "100 seizures a day!" She was on massive doses of anticonvulsants with no effect. Once on the program at the clinic the seizures slowed to only a few each day.

The child's mother was very receptive to this truth even though it was absolutely new to her understanding. We spoke often about the authority we have over all appearances of evil. Once while they were having an appointment at the clinic the child began to have a seizure. Immediately both the technician caring for the child and the mother said out loud, "No! I will not allow this!" Instantly the seizure stopped. Again about twenty minutes later she began to demonstrate signs that a seizure was about to begin and they repeated the same words. The seizure stopped before it really got started. For the first time in the life of the child she stopped having seizures, with no drugs! To date (this is only a few weeks later) there have been a few more occasions where she started to seize, but the words of authority spoken by the mother and now the rest of the family has stopped them every time. If they are consistent with this, and I know they will be, this manifestation of evil that has boastfully usurped authority over this child of God will be gone completely.

Another recent example of this principle is a woman with severely high blood sugar. She had unsuccessfully tried to control it with diet and exercise in the past and was disinclined to use drugs. She began to say "No!" to this manifestation of confusion and disorder whenever the blood sugar would elevate. And without exception it would instantly drop to normal! With consistency and dedication this also will be a distant memory.

So you see, no matter what or how darkness and confusion appears, no matter how long one has experienced it and no matter what the medical predictions, it is still only a suggestion, separate and apart from the Holy Son of God and we have a choice! We come with the fullness of God, and one of the attributes of that Nature is authority over all the works of darkness. We only need to use that authority...and mean it! This will silence once and for all the victim mentality and catapult us into our rightful inheritance and our right mind. We will cease to see these challenges as something real that needs to be healed and begin to realize that we are whole and intact as we have been formed…and these interruptions are but suggestions, external to us.

God has given us a choice. "Choose life or choose death." If we didn't have the ability to make the choice for life, this would have never been said. Isn't it time to believe God over the opinions and conclusions of mankind?

Remember that we are not ever a victim of anything, but always the Light and Power of God. When we make the separation from who we are and the influence of evil, we are strengthened to exercise our Power and Authority and be rid of it.

Sadly we are taught instead that God has a reason for our suffering. Or that we needed or deserved this suffering. Or that we are hereditarily inclined towards it. Any and all these words are the beginning of the enslavement to something we actually came to destroy!

Whatever it is, however it manifests on or in the body or mind, however long it has been around, however severe it may tell you it is, however severe others may believe it is…it is still *external suggestion of evil and you still have the authority to send it away.* Just say "No!" Just say "No!"

This is also true of any behavior problem, any "addiction," any manifestation of darkness. Just do it! Stay with it. "Do not be weary in well doing." This is the will and purpose of God for you in this situation. You have all of Eternity behind you and the words you speak.

Remember we were sent to "undo the works of darkness" and never to become a victim of them. We would not have been sent without the authority, strength, and dominion to remove them! We possess this authority! The words we speak are the power of God to every situation!

CHAPTER TEN

STAYING TRUE TO THE TRUTH

Once we have accepted who we are "in Christ" we must also accept this for everyone. This is not something we have earned, or had anything to do with at all. It is a fact of Creation. So everyone is included in this. "He is the true Light which lighteth every man born into the world. And of His fullness have we all received." We are not progressively coming into this fullness -- but possess it now and forever!

This drives people crazy who think that they had something to do with becoming the Holy Sons of God. They like to see themselves separate and apart from others who didn't do whatever they think they did to earn this state of being. It is the "we/ they" doctrine.

But the New Covenant was for all. "Behold! I will pour my Spirit out upon *all mankind*. I will cause them to know me...by my Spirit. They shall no longer say to one another, "Know the Lord, for *all shall know me* from the least to the greatest." And "Their sins (separated consciousness) and their iniquities I will remember no more."

～

There was a time, a moment in history when I released "my life" to God, who, I finally acknowledged, made me for His purpose, and not my own. At that moment I felt the Spirit of God filling my whole being and knew I was "a New Creature in Christ." I knew all the "old had passed away and all things were made new, and all things were from God," from that moment on and forever! I was, as Jesus put it, "Born of the Spirit." No doubt! But did that change what already was? Or was it that at that moment I suddenly was able to see, to know what had always been true? Nothing was changed. "Whatsoever God has made can not be added to or altered in any way." Instead I know now that I was awakened out from a terrible nightmare of separation and despair. I was able then to see what was *already established from before time began.* "For we were In Him from before the foundation of the world."

Why is this important? Because we must know that God is not doing anything to fix anything now. Everything is perfect as it is...it is only our perception, our understanding which needs to be awakened. The only change is *our seeing what is already*...the light shinning in the darkness. Otherwise we will find ourselves believing that God also looks upon this evil and acknowledges it as a power to overcome...and then may or may not "do something" in our behalf! It becomes a tug of war between good and evil...the way religion has for centuries presented it to us. Then we fall into *needing to earn* something or to qualify for our much needed healing. That then opens the door to failure, guilt and condemnation. No one can receive anything in that state!

But remember that God cannot be in the midst of such foolishness and still realize Himself as Eternal Omnipotence...the all and only Power. He would have not told us to stay away from serving other gods. (By acknowledging them as a power...thereby denying God as the only Power.)

And above all this He would not have told us that "in the day we partake of the (constant war between) good and evil, we would surely die!" Instead He declared to us that the only partaking we would be able to do *to live* was to "Eat (partake) of the knowledge of One Life only." (And we all a manifestation of it!) It may be good here to read the 17th chapter of the book of John and see for yourself what was the prayer, the burning desire of Jesus for us, if not to come to this understanding once and for all!

So now we know everyone is a part of the Son of God...whether they see, know or acknowledge this or not. They may be the worst in terms of human behavior. They may be manifesting the lowest, most depraved behavior, but nothing changes this Eternal fact. Sin is sin. It is all "separation from the knowledge of our true identity." *It is in connecting with the knowledge of our true identity* that sin, or a sense of being separated from Eternal Life, is removed. So the idea is not to condemn and desire punishment...but to realize we are the Son(s) of God, sent here for the Eternal Purpose of awakening Creation to its present wholeness and perfection. We desire "the earth to be filled with the knowledge of the Lord as the waters cover the sea."

ॐ

The way we approach someone in need of healing or more correctly put, *awakening*, is to not impute iniquity, not judge, not condemn, not try to correct or change anything, not try to convince them of truth, but to *see their present reality clearly ourselves.* To see beyond the appearance to *that which never changes.* To see the "Glory of God in the face of Jesus Christ." To see the Holy Son of God in all his radiant Glory…right where the sinning, sick mortal is appearing. How do we do this? By making the separation.

Realize first we are dealing with a *thought* that has attached itself to this sleeping Son of God. We separate the thought from the individual. The thought is what is appearing here. And the thought is darkness, ignorance of truth. So we separate one from the other. We *send away the offending thought*…and it must go in response to your word…and then *lift up the Christ,* the Holy Son. I then speak to this Christ, this Son, words of truth. I do this in my mind only. I tell it that it is Love itself. It is Life itself. It is Eternal and Beloved of the Father. I remind it of its present Glory and wholeness. I may even take its hand and embrace it. From the time I send away the offending darkness, I don't look at it again. My whole focus is on the Son of God and reminding it who it is and why it is. No matter how long it takes, I stay with it till the desired results are obtained. And the desired result is the full awakening of the consciousness of the individual…never stopping with simply a reversal in symptoms or improved behavior. That would invite the thought back at some other time. However if the individual is truly awakened to his Eternal identity, he knows then why he can live above this conflict and will not allow it a future existence.

This is as easily done with oneself as it is with another. King David spoke to his own soul when he told it to "Be still" reminding it that "The Lord has dealt bountifully with thee." So we may just as simply heal ourselves, or awaken ourselves, as we *must* do for others.

Healing is just that simple. The work is done within our own souls, daily, hourly. Every time darkness rears its ugly head we must never capitulate, never acquiesce to its suggestions of authority and power, but in every case remember the Omnipotence of Omnipresence.

CHAPTER ELEVEN

AN EXAMPLE OF
HEALING BY REPENTANCE

Recently I was asked to pray for a situation where a very young child, who had been previously diagnosed with a malignant brain tumor, was now scheduled for another craniotomy because an MRI had revealed that the tumor had returned. Specifically I was asked to pray that the MRI which was to be done just before the surgery would turn up negative.

Understandably the family was frantic, but I knew that .praying in this manner would only leave them vulnerable to the next negative report. The answer was to lift their consciousness above the whole terrifying mess into the place where God is good and God is all that is. To lift them to the place where "nothing shall by any means hurt you." To lift them to the place where this lying threat was finished once and forever.

To pray for the test results to be favorable is still to believe in the validity of the test results in the first place. It is placing one's trust in the tests rather than in the absolute truth…in spite of the tests. I spoke to the caller about this and she seemed to understand the words but clearly had no idea how to get to that place in her heart. I told her I would pray.

I always begin by specifically asking the Holy Spirit for guidance in how to proceed in prayer. I know that the Spirit "searches the hearts" of those involved and knows what they need, what they are holding in their thought which would block the healing and exactly how to allow the flow of light, life and power to be experienced.

I had recently heard of a Hawaiian healing prayer, a formula for healing, so to speak, and I was moved by the beauty and simplicity of it. My understanding of it is probably quite different from the original, but I worked with what I knew. It is simply to look at the person needing the healing (in your mind) and say "I am so sorry!" "Please forgive me!" "I love you!" and finally, "Thank you." I want to break this down for you as I see it in my heart.

I am so sorry says to me, "I am so sorry for what we have believed about you. We are the Holy Sons of God, sent here to heal and to see truth and beauty and wholeness everywhere and we have instead believed this horrible stuff and attached it to you, causing you great suffering. I am so sorry we didn't know this. I am so sorry we did not see your intrinsic wholeness and beauty. I am so sorry we, (as a many membered, yet ONE son), have failed you. Please forgive me."

Now I stood in the place of the whole son and said, "I love you and I will prove my love for you by choosing to see only truth. I will prove my love for you by sending away this whole ugly lie about you, who is forever made in the radiance of God only."

At this point I begin to repent for all the horror that was ever said, done, believed, repeated, and written concerning this particular disease. I repented in behalf of every person who ever lived that even just once gave power to this horror in their lives. Even those who made drugs or treatment to deal with it. Anyone who ever mentioned it, suffered because of the belief, or in any way dealt with it. I called it a strange god, idolatry, a non-power. I released it from every soul, leaving the whole Son of God free to see this child whole and perfect.

I spoke to the child, telling him of his true identity, his Divine Purpose for being here and the Eternal Shepherd's unending Love and care for him. I saw that there was only One Mind, One Divine influence governing all of Creation. Therefore all creation, including him, was certainly maintained in uninterrupted Divine Order.

A week later I received a letter from the one who originally called me for prayer. She had in essence done the same thing herself. She repeated to me the prayer that she said and in it she agreed to his perfection, his beauty and his wholeness. She gave no power to the appearance and "magnified the God of Life, beauty and grace." Needless to say, the tests were negative, the surgery was avoided and more than anything else, the family realized a lasting peace and a future without fear for the child. They came into the knowledge of the truth in spades!

This is an example of the power of releasing the soul

from the insanity that covers it. This is only one story, but there are thousands more. The value of clearing the way for the ever-present Glory of God to appear cannot be repeated enough. This is the simplicity of healing.

CHAPTER TWELVE

HOW DO WE PRAY FOR THOSE WHO DO NOT OR CAN NOT PRAY FOR THEMSELVES?

A close acquaintance of mine received a diagnoses of prostate cancer. He was pretty much unenlightened spiritually but still believed that I could heal him and asked for my help. He was not inclined to submit his body to the medical route. I tried unsuccessfully to encourage him to begin to "press into his spiritual nature," develop a relationship with God, and learn of the faithfulness and Mercy of God and the absoluteness of the truth of his intact spiritual being. He dabbled at it but was basically disinterested.

As the months passed and his fear elevated, he became more withdrawn, angry and oftentimes overtly belligerent. Finally he announced that he was going to the doctor. He asked if I would accompany him and I agreed.

Once there, many tests were done and each one confirmed a "large malignant growth on the left lobe of the prostate gland." He was scheduled for further tests the following week.

Several days later while I was driving to work I became

frustrated with the whole scenario. I wondered how to heal someone who is unconsciously resisting the Spirit and Power of the truth. Then it came to me to repent in his behalf. I remember just repenting for his whole life being lived without the Spirit of God being allowed to direct and possess it. It was a kind of blanket covering of it all. And suddenly, right in the middle of a sentence, I realized a virtual explosion of Life as it filled my car. I looked out the window at every manifestation of Life now a brilliant, almost iridescent green. My heart soared and I knew he was healed. And he was. Never again was there any indication of affliction, no matter the extensive testing that they continued to do.

My experience with this kind of healing is that since the consciousness remained that allowed the affliction in the first place, those folks go on to other experiences of disease or worse. In my first book, "Of Monkeys and Dragons, Freedom from the Tyranny of Disease," I told two stories of men who were healed from heart disease and colon cancer. Neither one was aware of any degree of truth and therefore the thoughts and beliefs remained unchanged. Both were later killed in car accidents. This was my earliest understanding that the mind, the belief, was the source and the body only the affect. It was somewhat discouraging because I knew that while I was able to heal a *manifestation* of belief, I never penetrated the consciousness of the individuals. A true healing is one of the heart, the understanding. That would have to come later for my friend.

With every experience we face we have a choice to deal with it spiritually or not. If we choose to deal with an event

on a spiritual level we will pray to know what new understanding is waiting for us to learn. We will ask the heart of
Wisdom to reveal to us a truth, an understanding that we
were not aware of before. And when it comes, the healing
will follow. The wonderful thing about this is that once a
healing comes as a result of a new understanding, it is a
permanent healing, forever throughout eternity! The truth
shall make you free!

And now a note about our children: We are the covering, the blanket of protection for them so long as they are
children. They are blessed according to the consciousness
we hold. Conversely, when our thoughts are unenlightened,
or we are holding some untruth in our atmosphere of
thought, our lives project confusion and we unknowingly,
unconsciously allow darkness to rule our affairs. Often chaos
and confusion is allowed to creep into their lives as well.

When people come for prayer concerning their children,
my thoughts and my attention is always directed to the
consciousness of the parents, or those who cover them. I
deal with the thoughts of the doctors and the extended family members as well. As the truth of One Mind is applied to
the situation, fear, hysteria, despair and the like are sub-
dued by a sense of peace, confidence and an expectation of
goodness. Then the child is healed.

Once again though the basic understanding of those
covering the children will either be corrected or remain the
same. If there is no new understanding or elevation of consciousness from a particular event, another challenge will
most certainly occur.

Most of you know that my second child was born with severe and innumerable physical problems that were expected to either take her life or destroy any opportunity for a normal life. This was a direct reflection of the disjointed confusion of my life and my thoughts at that time. As I began to turn my attention wholeheartedly to God, my mind and my emotions, my understanding and my peace began to be establish according to truth. *With no other influence,* she was healed and remains so to this day.

Now the day will come in the life of the child, as he becomes an adult, when he must search out his own thoughts and choose his own path of understanding. At that point he is no longer under the umbrella of the understanding of his parents, but responsible for his own choices of thought.

Should we pray for those adults who don't pray for themselves, who don't search for truth and understanding? As we are led by the Spirit of God, we should. Who knows what experience will finally turn them to the heart of God, even as we were turned.

Remember we are not healing a person so much as we are declaring what is true and what is false. We are choosing to honor the truth of the Omnipotence of One God only and give no power to evil imaginations. We are here to bring the Light of truth to a very confused and convoluted world thought and every opportunity that is presented to us is opportunity to do just that.

CHAPTER THIRTEEN

RELEASING THE POWER OF GOD

When it's all said and done...when all the books have been read and all the truths have been known...when we have gone to every meeting and have 'workshopities'. Still it comes down to releasing the Spirit of Power that resides within us. It is the *flow* of this that brings the power needed for the correction or healing we seek.

The truth is we don't need to know anything at all to experience the release of the Spirit. It doesn't flow by any amount of "head knowledge" we have accumulated. I have found that we only need to sing! We only need to praise and exalt the Presence of the Lord.

The name "Lord" refers to the Power, the authority, the dominion and strength over *every* and *all* suggestions of evil. Darkness, all forms of evil appearances, can declare whatever power it wants us to think it has...but it knows that there is only One Power! The key is that *we* also need to know this is true. When we are hit with a manifestation of evil that stops us in our tracks, it is sometimes difficult to get to where we need to be spiritually.

When we begin to sing, to lift up the "name of the Lord," as Psalms directs us to do, we are declaring that all power belongs to good. All power belongs to God. We are declaring where we have chosen to put our confidence. The Bible calls this "offering the sacrifice of thanksgiving unto God." If you have ever tried to sing and worship the "name of the Lord" in the midst of a crises, you will know why it is called a sacrifice. It is difficult to turn our attention away from the apparent threat. But this is exactly what needs to be done. We cannot panic, worry, fret, run screaming down the road… and be worshipping and singing at the same time. When we decide to sing, to praise, we are taking a stand against evil. When our heart is pounding in our chest, this is the time to sing the loudest!

Recently I was facing an ugly attitude, a judgment, a condemning spirit acting through someone who was ignorant that he was being used by evil. I thought about defending myself. I thought about declaring my innocence. I thought about how wrong he was. But then I thought about the Power of God. Then I thought about how much power I was giving to darkness. So I began to sing. I sang at the top of my lungs and as I sang I was amazed to find how much power I was feeling. I was amazed at the sudden turn of power and control. Instead of the events ruling my heart… strength and power, dominion and authority began to rule my heart. I could feel the darkness dissipating! I never uttered a word of prayer. The song of praise was all the prayer I needed. Later in the day I began to understand the voice of

Wisdom speaking to my heart. Constructive direction mingled with confidence was the dominating spirit. The situation was unable to rule my heart again!

We are either thinking, ruminating, analyzing, problem solving or better, problem worrying...or we are singing. We are either trying to fix it ourselves or making a deliberate choice to know Divine Power is always governing in Order, harmony, Wisdom, beauty and perfection. This is surrender. We are not outlining, trying to direct God, feeling the need to inform God, asking for God to fix it...we are *knowing* Omnipotence is Omnipresent! We are declaring, choosing and meaning it when we say, "As in heaven, so shall your will be done on earth." Your Life, your Wisdom, your Presence will be revealed right here, right now. This is trusting. This is absolute surrender. People always ask how to surrender. This is it!

Let's look at some of the stories in the Bible concerning this topic. Remember that these are documented for our example.

IIChronicles chapter 20:

Jehoshaphat was a godly and righteous King who served God in humility and obedience. When a siege of enemy nations came against them Jehoshaphat sought the Wisdom and counsel of God. He was instructed to set his army in order for battle but was comforted with the words, "You shall not have to fight this battle, for I will fight it for you." Further he was instructed to send the singers, musicians and all those who praised the Lord with music out in front of the army. They were to sing and praise and shout in joy and gladness to the Lord...right in the line of fire! And they willingly did just that. The confusion of the attacking army was so great they began to slaughter each other and Jehoshaphat's army was spared to the last man. Not an arrow was shot. Not a sword was drawn. They sang their way to victory.

Joshua chapter 6:

Joshua led the entire nation of Israel into the Promised Land after the death of Moses. He had a pure and fervent heart towards God and he was a man of conviction and faith. After crossing Jordon they came to one last obstacle before entering into the land, the city of Jericho. It was well fortified, surrounded by great and mighty walls of protection. Joshua was such a strong man of conviction, dedication and prayer, that instead of driving the Israelite army head on into the city, he prayed and received this instruction. He was to have the singers and musicians lead the nation as they surrounded the Jericho wall. They were to quietly march, once a day for seven days, around the city. On the seventh day they were to shout with a loud shout unto the Lord. They sang and played their instruments with all their hearts. At this point the walls came down before them causing great confusion for the city of Jericho. They were able to scale the fallen walls and take the city with little to no resistance.

Jonah chapter 2

Jonah was told by God to go to a city called Nineveh, whose inhabitants had turned their hearts away from the Lord. He was to tell them to repent because great evil was coming to them. God wanted to show them Mercy but Jonah wanted them to suffer for their sins. He was angry that God had Mercy for them…when he, himself, was a righteous man and thought they should not be blessed unless they also lived righteously. So he ran from his instruction and landed in the "belly of hell," depicted as a great whale. "I cried by reason of my affliction unto the Lord and He heard me. Out of the belly of hell cried I and thou heard my voice." And here is the classic line. "Those that observe lying vanities forsake their own mercies." In other words, those who focus on the problem, which is a "lying vanity" according to God, *actually block the very solution to their problem.* Those that focus on what they may have done to cause this problem or what must be done humanly to solve it…all this is part of the "lying vanity." The focus must be on the goodness of God, on the ever present Mercy of God. The focus must be on the Eternal constant Love of God, His Power and strength and His fervent protection from any harm. No matter that it was "his fault" that he was in this mess. He knew the Mercy of God poured out goodness *in spite* of human behavior!

We cannot be singing and praising and worrying and doubting at the same time! We cannot be reflecting on the covering protection of God (even if we think we have "deserved" this problem) and be fretting at the same time. Jonah went on the say, "I offered a sacrifice of thanksgiving and the Lord heard me and caused the fish to spit me out on dry land." Needless to say he finally did as he was told and everything turned out well. But the point is that in the midst of hell, he moved in a spirit of thanksgiving, knowing the Mercy of God was everlasting. All he needed to do was to activate the flow. Even in his disobedience he expected

Mercy and got it! "Behold, if I make my bed in hell, Thou are with me."

Acts chapter 16:

The Apostle Paul and his companion Silas found themselves in Jail for preaching the words and person of Jesus to certain people who made their living serving false gods. Instead of considering the unfairness of their plight, they began to sing and praise God at *the midnight hour.* The darkest time of their imprisonment, the most desperate hour of their soul. They sang and rejoiced loud enough for everyone to hear. Not coincidently, an earthquake caused the prison doors to open for all the prisoners to be free. So great was their soul freed by song! So great was the Power and Presence released by their song and worship.

IISamuel chapter 6:

*My very favorite is the s*tory of David, who shortly after being crowned King of all Israel, determined to return the Arc of the Covenant to Jerusalem. You might remember that the Arc of the Covenant represented the very Presence and Power of God to the Israelites. It is full of symbolism for us today, but sufficient for now the Arc was lost in battle by the disobedience of Saul, the preceding king. David knew he must return it to his people if they were to ever enjoy the goodness and protection of God. So off he marched. Regaining the Arc was not difficult but transporting it back to Jerusalem proved to be the challenge.

At one point the oxen that pulled the cart upon which the Arc rested stumbled, causing the Arc to rock in an unsteady manner. One of the priests reached out to steady it and as he touched it he suddenly died!

You see, under no condition was this Arc to be touched by human hands. Signifying that this whole mortal time for us here on earth is to be performed by the Wisdom and Power of God. When we "run ahead" of God in a matter... not inquiring, receiving or following Divine direction... we are, in effect, touching the Arc. If there is one lesson to be learned for us in this whole lifetime it is this. Life will go well when we begin to let God lead. When we realize *who* this Life called "me" truly is and who is responsible for it. This is true submission and humility. This is the nature of the Lamb of God. A nature willing to let its Shepherd lead, trusting all will be well.

Once David figured out that he needed to stop in his pursuit of bringing the Arc home and take the time to pray and ask for direction, all went much better. You see, his desire was good and noble, but Wisdom has Its way to fulfill desires and needs.

Again the instruction came to place the singers, and all those who worship with instruments of music out in front of the entourage, leading the Arc back home. "Shouting, singing, dancing and making loud and joyful 'noise' to God."

Now the question might come to your mind, "Does God need this?" And the answer is "No, we do!" We need to clear all thoughts, all efforts, all fears, all doubts...anything and everything which would block the free and easy flow of the Spirit of Power and dominion through us. The way to this is the sacrifice of praise and thanksgiving.

In Philippians, chapter 4, verses 6 and 7 we read, *"Be*

anxious for nothing. In *everything* by prayer and supplication, *with thanksgiving*, make your requests known unto the Lord and the God of peace will keep your hearts and minds through Christ Jesus."

The Psalms, particularly the second half, are filled with the clear instruction to praise, worship and thank God for His great and wonderful Mercy. This is how we are made ready to receive Mercy in times of need.

If this is new to you and you feel hesitant, go into a room alone, pretend someone just gave you several million dollars and let yourself act out the joy you would feel. How would you feel if this problem you carry were completely gone? Act now as if it is, and it will be. Don't be inhibited, be inhabited... by joy and gladness. It is worth far more than all the riches and all the health and all the happiness the world can offer you.

CHAPTER FOURTEEN

IN HIM

"In Him we live and move and have our being." What does it mean to be "in Him?"

Ephesians says we have been "in Him from before the foundation of the world." Colossians tells us that we are "complete in Him." Further it says we are "seated at the right hand of the power of God, in Him." In Him we experienced baptism when Jesus did. In Him we experienced death, burial and resurrection when Jesus did, making us free from these dreadful experiences in that we have already "been there and done that!" And therefore death can hold us no more! This is the hope we have "in Him," but what does it mean exactly?

The 'Him' referred to is the Spirit of God and that Spirit is Life and that Spirit is Love and that Spirit is Light. God is not a Being who loves, but Love Itself. God is not a Being who imparts Life, but Life Itself. God does not shine forth the Light, but is the Light Itself. We are *in that Life and in that Love and in that Light from before the worlds were formed.* Job says that "The Sons of God shouted for joy in the Presence of God before ever the worlds were formed!" Nothing can change that...nothing we do, nothing we think, nothing we know or don't know. It is an Eternal fact of being. We live in Him. We don't have to get there, earn it, seek it or pray for it to be. It simply is. For those of you who are devoted disciples of the Bible, this is the "mystery of God" referred to by Paul again and again in the book of Ephesians. This is also the fulfillment of the prayer spoken by Jesus, in John, chapter 17.

Therefore we *are not in this present situation* even as it appears...we are in Him instead. We cannot be in both light and darkness. We must choose...not based on what is appearing ("While we look not at those things which are seen but to those things which are unseen.")

We are not living in a body, as we have believed. Life goes on long after the body. No, we are, have always been and will always be, in Him. By choosing to confess and hold to this truth we honor God who is the Truth. We fulfill our purpose for being here. We declare the Kingdom of God is Omnipresent and Omnipotent. This drives away all appearances of darkness, evil and confusion. The honoring this...the knowing this and sticking to it in spite of the present appearances, will be our healing.

We live in the air that surrounds us, don't we? That air is referred to as "pneumo." It also means breath, and Spirit. We don't see the air with our eyes, and yet we live in it. We don't see Him, the Life and Love and Light, and yet we live in it as well.

This is the Kingdom of God that Jesus spoke of when He said it was here and all around us, not far off and needing to be reached or earned. He said it was "in us" and we were in it.

We enter into the conscious realization of this by a simple act of repentance. Repentance means to *choose* to turn towards another way, another thought, another belief.

"Repent, for the Kingdom of God (government, rule and reign) of God is at hand." By this it is meant that we choose to turn towards the realization of it, leaving behind all the confusion and darkness of mortal thinking. We can do this right now.

We simply close our eyes to shut out the visible world and all its distractions. We breathe in deeply the Spirit of Life and we just as deeply exhale the clutter of the world. We do this several times and then become very still. In this stillness we feel the intensity of Love surrounding us. We feel this for several minutes and then we feel the Life flowing through us, electrifying and powerful. Contained within this Life are all the attributes of Perfection, wholeness and harmony. It is uninterrupted Eternal Order and *nothing has the capacity to interfere.* It is full and abundant. As it flows through us it finds a source of complete expression. We remain still and we allow it to manifest itself however it chooses without our thoughts or our influence. We know it is Wisdom and we trust this Eternal Wisdom. We surrender to Wisdom, to Life and we surrender to Love. This Love is our Shepherd. It leads and guides, covers and protects, feeds and clothes us. It takes care of us. It takes care of those we love. It takes care of our business, our bodies, our homes, our world. It is the Life of all this and so much more. We let it be who it is. We let it flow.

In Him nothing can hurt us. Nothing can reach us. Many things will threaten and declare its power to hurt us, but in spite of the clamor of multitudes of threats, nothing can reach us in Him. All powers and fears dissolve and fade away as we hold ourselves in the conscious awareness of being in Him. We can face anything that appears in this world of many appearances, and as we hold to this truth nothing can reach us.

In Him also refers to being in the conscious realization of our true identity. We have for so long been immersed into the idea of mortality, with a beginning and an end. We have for so long felt vulnerable to the world we have been sent to. We have adopted an attitude of frailty and weakness, a "victim mentality" to the "law" of chance, the roll of the dice kind of living, ducking the blows around every corner, never knowing what may come to hurt or interrupt our lives next. We have believed that the highest conscious thought relating to God is that we use Him to fix us.

In all this confusion we have forgotten why we were sent here and who we were. Instead we adopted the very same confusion and insanity found in the darkness of the minds of men that we were sent to awaken.

We have a continual choice here when faced with any appearance of lack, limitation, disease, discord or threat of any kind. The choice is *where do we live*? Do we live in a world of fear, change and vulnerability, needing God to fix every situation we find ourselves immersed into? Or do we stand strong in the face of anything that declares its ability to cause us harm and declare that we are "in Him" and therefore a "target out of reach!" Are we still considering our various *options* in any situation or are we denying the ability of anything to hurt or interrupt us to start with. *Where do we live?* In the mortal, with all of its problems or in the safety and uninterrupted security of being forever *in Him?*

In all this confusion we read the words of Paul who said that the day must come when we, who saw ourselves as mortals, must "take on the realization of immorality." We, who saw ourselves as corruptible, must "take on the realization of incorruptibility." We must find our selves immersed in Him. We must learn from our teacher, the Holy Spirit of God, sent to "lead and guide us into all truth" how to live as the Holy Son (expression) of God. We must learn how to hear His Voice and step out in confidence and assurance. The kind of confidence and assurance that comes with knowing you are His Light, and the Love of His Life, sent to dissolve darkness of every sort.

This is not something man can take unto himself. That is, we cannot, with the pride of man, simply declare this and in our pitiful arrogance think we can, by saying it, manifest it. This is something that God *by grace alone* reveals to us. It produces a deep sense of humility and devotion to the Love and Life that sent us here. It causes us to desire to live to fulfill His purpose and not to live to satisfy our own shallow wants and desires. It breaks through the stony ground of the souls of men and reveals the soft and powerful heart of God bursting forth from within. It dissolves all fears and evil imaginations and we begin to know…

To find our true Life we must give our pitiful idea of "my life" to God to break through and let Life flow. We cannot cling to our idea of life and ever expect to be immersed into the Life that is In Him.

John, chapter 16 finds Jesus sharing with his disciples the transition from being outside of Him and asking for things, asking for help, asking for whatever we need…which He is more than happy to give, by the way…and finally being in such a state of *knowing* our inherent Oneness with Him that we will need to ask nothing and yet live in the goodness of all things.

To get to this awareness, simply desire it and stay with that desire more than any other thought you entertain. Know that it is by grace alone. Know that it is the ultimate will of God for each one of us. Know that it will come to pass. And never try to make it happen by empty words or strange human ways and means. Just trust.

❧ GOD IS
ETERNAL SOUL

What is the soul? In my mind it is the *expression* of a life. It is how *who we think we are* is expressed and manifested. We express how we see ourselves. Do we see ourselves as victims of disease? As criminals? As addicts? As abandoned?

Right now we see individual souls and therefore individual expressions. But for a moment realize that there is really only one Life and that Life is expressing Itself as each one individually and as all of us collectively. It expresses itself as all of Creation as well. God is that One Life. Everywhere we look we see God *expressing Himself as, in and through, all that is made visible, including you and me.* God is the Eternal Soul of Man. This is a good description of the Son of God...the collective, visible expression of the invisible God. Think of it for a moment. Imagine that everything and everyone you look at is actually God or Eternal Life expressing Itself. As we choose to see this we choose to see God instead of merely things, or people. With this foremost in our minds, that which we look upon begins to take on the beauty and perfection of the One who lives in and through it. II Corinthians says " I am determined to know no man after the flesh: yea, though I have known Jesus after the flesh -- I will know Him no more." But all men as reflections of the spirit and manifestation of Eternal Life.

In I Corinthians, chapter 15 we read "The first man, Adam, was a living soul. The last Adam is a life giving Spirit." We understand that the same Spirit that manifested through and as Jesus is now residing within us, as the very Spirit of our life. This is the basis of our Oneness. So there is only One Son, the "only begotten son" and we are all one in Him.

So if Jesus is the LAST Adam, what about all of us? The answer is we are all "in Him." "Hid in Christ in God."

We know that it is not speaking of a single person when it says the "first Adam." The first Adam is speaking of the whole of the mortal identity. The "old man" as the Bible

calls it...or the "carnal man." This is the Adamic consciousness that brought sin (separation from who we are) into the
world. It is the world thought! It is lost in confusion...so
lost it doesn't even know it is lost! So also the "last Adam"
is not only referring to one, but all *as that one*.

Now comes the revealing or appearing of the true
man...the spiritual man...the One who we all are. As the
first man, Adam is a collective man, so is the many-mem-
bered, collective son of God. Right out from the midst of
the darkness of the *first man* comes the Son. Out from under the rubble of the destruction of the old comes forth the
new. And this is how it will always appear...right out from
the midst of you and me. Out from the grave of our own
mortal thinking, the Christ will appear.

This is the "last Adam." It was revealed to the earth by
Jesus...but is He the last and therefore the only Son? Yes!
And this point is critical to all healings. There is only one
Son and we are all "in Him" as one Divine Being. When we
realize that we are not dealing with this individual or that,
but the One and only Son...we will see the world healed
and every person a part of that healing. We will understand
the powerlessness of any other voice. When Mother Theresa
was asked how she was able to care for the sick and poor
and wretched of India, she was often quoted as saying, "I
see the face of Jesus in many suffering souls."

We must, must make the separation between the old
man, the one who believes he is sick, believes he is poor,
believes he is a victim, the one who is so abusive and sin-

ful, the one who the whole world hates… and the Son. Generations of dealing with the mortal, the first man, Adam, ought to tell us that this is not the way to heal anything. Sin, sickness and death still run rampant in the earth. For all our efforts on the human level, *dealing with the problem as it appears, with all the failures to heal or to sustain permanent healings… ought to tell us that there is a better way!*

This bears repeating again and again…make the separation! See the offending condition "outside" of you (or whoever you are healing.) Never see the offending disease or sin as originating from within. We have the Mind of Christ. One mind, not two minds. This mind could never conceive darkness. No, all evil is an external thought, a suggestion of a power other than God (other than you as the soul of God.) once you see it separate from you or another, release it! Repent of ever having listened to it and given it your consent. Not with a sorrowful, heavy heart as one who is guilty. But with a deliberate, firm authority. Send it away! Then all that remains is a space to be filled with the Light and Glory of the Son!

When you know you are in touch with the Son…you can draw Him forth. You can strengthen Him, exalt Him, speak the truth to Him to lift Him up, cover His nakedness…his sin… and feed Him with love and devotion. He will… before your eyes… become stronger, more visible, until finally He will arise in all His fullness and Glory and there will be a healing unlike anything you have ever expected!

∂

Bless the Son. Psalms says "Kiss the Son." But always remember that you are speaking to the Son deep within the person or persons you are praying for. The same Son who lived and left 2000 years ago. You see, he never left! He said "I will be with you always, even to the ends of the earth." He will be with us because He is the Life of each one of us! He is our real and only Life! His Spirit is the very Spirit of our Life. He is the last, the all, the only Son...the expression of God...or the soul of God. He is our true identity.

So God's soul is the Son, the visible expression of Himself and of all Creation! This is how He expresses Life and Glory and beauty and completion in and to the earth.

The awareness of this brings healings and brings Life. Learn to see everyone as the soul of God. Your life will be healed and so will the lives of all you meet. You will be fulfilling the reason you were sent here. This is what it's all about and how it all happens. This is "God, all and in all." This is what the world awaits to see...and to be.

CHAPTER FIFTEEN

FROM SERVANT TO SON

"The servant knows not what the Master of the household does, but the son knows."

There is a progressive unfolding of conscious understanding and expression of the Christ consciousness. We generally begin as one who feels separate and apart from God and believe our whole purpose is to win His favor and thereby gain a better life here, as well as heaven hereafter. This, of course, speaks of a God of reward and punishment. This was the understanding of God as revealed by the Old Testament, but re-introduced by Jesus as *not exacting punishment* for transgressions, but only dealing in Mercy and Grace.

Hopefully we progress beyond that thought and begin to realize that "The Father and I are one." Once "oneness" has dawned upon us and awakened us to know that we have nothing to gain or earn for we possess all that God is...and that we are not rewarded or punished (except as we believe it to be so)... but exist as the embodied beloved of the Father...the source of all Life, we then can begin to "be about our Father's business." We want to fulfill our Divine Purpose and no longer live to serve ourselves, for it is in this thought only that we can find joy and peace and a wonderful sense of fulfillment.

But how do we make this transition? Basically we are asking, "How do we move out from the mortal thought, with all of its victimhood and suffering, into the reality of immortality? How do we make the shift from the corruptible to the incorruptible? How do we *live out* from being one with the Father? How do we be the Sons of God? How do we get there?"

Of course the complete answer is that God does it by the working of the Spirit...which is called grace. But we do have an action in all this...a cooperative action that merely "speaking words" will not accomplish.

We all want to make this new spiritual understanding happen in our lives. Unfortunately we do some pretty strange things sometimes to try to facilitate this. We waste a lot of time and effort trying things instead of simply *asking* our Father for the needed direction. We listen to the "wisdom of men," of which Jesus said, "You make the commandments (ways) of God of none effect by your traditions and doctrines." Soon enough we realize that the "wisdom of men" is no wisdom at all.

We read where people, just like you and me, would engage in prolonged fasting, walking or kneeling for days, weeks. We read where they sometimes beat themselves, thinking that producing pain would put their bodies under subjection to the Spirit, thereby producing the desired "oneness" with God.

These days we engage in religious rituals such as lighting candles, attending services, saying certain prayers, frequent baptisms, many "alter calls" and the like. Some folks beat drums, change their names to reflect the names of others who have, in their minds, attained what they wish for themselves. All this is an effort to "make it happen." While these may be helpful on some level, yet there is a better way.

Everyone has things in their lives that they would like improvement on, such as their jobs, their finances, their health, their families, etc. Some would like to find a meaningful relationship, some have a life-long dream they wish would come to fruition. But whatever it is we dream of, we must come to understand that it is all available within our relationship to our Creator. Only how to access that seems to be the stumbling block.

We know that God has and is the power to make things happen. We know that He has entrusted that power to us. Yet for all this knowledge, we still remain in the position of lack or limitation. How do we reconcile this?

Obviously the bongo drums, the endless walking through the labyrinths, the many alter calls, etc. have not brought this about. So our ways and means have failed and we need to know where to turn next.

To me the way is clear as I read the account of the Life and words of Jesus as recorded in the book of John. There has never been one who so clearly grasped the Life and Power of God as Jesus. There has never been one who so clearly utilized what was always available to mankind and who was so very successful in his efforts as Jesus. And of all the writings about the Life of this one, none so clearly defines the way to attain this in our own lives as John, the beloved disciple. The others told the story. But this one showed us the "how to." He alone grasped the words and the depth of the import of those words.

Jesus came not only to love and heal mankind from the darkness that had entombed them. He came to deliver to us the key to the Kingdom of God...right here and now. He came declaring that this Kingdom (the place of dominion and authority of perpetual goodness, everything we needed and must have to live victoriously and abundantly,) was already here among us, within us and easily accessible to us. He refuted the notion that we must somehow earn it, die to attain to it, or any of the other religious notions embraced for so long. He told us how, he showed us how, and he did it himself, that we might easily follow the way. He was in all points the "Good Shepherd," leading us into green pastures and restoring our souls. He still is.

Basically he taught us that the way to gain is to be willing to lose. The way *up* is to be willing to go down. He who exalts himself shall be humbled, but he who humbles himself shall be exalted. To cling to our lives is to lose our lives, but to fully yield our lives to another is to gain our life. We gain by giving. We lose by clinging.

In John chapter 12 there were two Greeks who came seeking Jesus. They asked to "see him." Jesus understood that they wanted more than to see him with their eyes, but to really see what made him who he was, able to do and speak and attain to that which mankind has sought for centuries. So he encapsulated all the longing and confusion and misunderstanding of the ages into one answer.

"Tell them that unless they are willing to lose their lives they will never gain what they seek. But if they are willing to *deny themselves,* they shall find themselves."

So churches read that, and not understanding the meaning, they began to impose restrictions upon their members, believing that those restrictions were the answer to "denying themselves." That of course never produced the desired results.

Paul said later, "I die daily." He further said that his life was "not his own" but belonged to Him who made him. And this is the key.

He saw Life as *someone rather than something.* He saw he was a created being *sent* to this realm of darkness to perform a purpose and not to serve himself, his life, his personal gain. He saw his life *absorbed in the one great Life* and he, himself, here to *serve* that one great Life and His holy purpose. He realized he was not a possessor of his life. As a matter of fact he had an uncanny detachment to having a personal life and instead saw himself only as an *extension of this one Life.* He lived to fulfill its purpose and was persuaded that it was to prove that power, might and dominion belong to God and God was only *good.* He taught that the kingdom of God was here, was good, and the result of yielding to it was always going to yield Life to the one surrendering to it.

The most disturbing phenomena I have encountered is what I have named as "the spiritual butterfly syndrome." This is reserved for folks who flit from here to there accumulating truths and spiritual information but never really applying what they are hearing. They are content to attend meetings after meetings enjoying what they hear, but it doesn't seem to take root in their souls.

Jesus spoke of these folks when he told the story of the man who built his house upon the sand. When the winds and the storms of life come the house is swept away for it lacked foundation. Conversely the man who built his house upon the rock (Truth) was able to withstand the storms that appeared. He finishes his parable with a challenge, "Be ye therefore a doer of the word and not a hearer only!"

Earlier Jesus told a parable of a farmer who went out to sow his seeds. "Some fell on rocks, some fell on thorns and thistles and some fell on good soil." When asked for clarification, Jesus said that the rocks were the hearts too hard to receive, the thorns and thistles were the cares of the world that choked out the new life...but those that fell on good soil were those who heard the word and "kept it."

Recently I spoke with a man about this and I said that it would be more beneficial for us to know only one truth and be faithful to use it when faced with evil suggestions and appearances than to have accumulated bags of truths and understandings and not apply them. "To whom much is given, much is required!"

The answer is in loving the "Lord your God with all your heart, soul, mind and strength." We do this by yielding our desires, our dreams, our wants and even our needs to him who is perfectly able to bless those and give us the increase. But first we must "let it go." Stop clinging to the way it needs to appear...or when. When we really love we trust the one we embrace. If we don't trust, we are in fear...whether our hearts are pounding in anxiety or not...it is still fear. The opposite of love is fear.

One thing that enables me to trust and to love in the face of sometimes horrible circumstances, is that I walk alone, for hours if necessary, and I choose to walk surrounding myself with nature. I remember that God is Life and therefore the very Life of everything formed. I begin to *feel* what I am seeing instead of just seeing it. I *listen* for sounds that creatures make, specifically different from all others. I believe that I am feeling and listening to the very Life of it all. I leave the human horror behind and I remember God as Life. If the Life of everything, then also that which holds it all together and in Divine Order. As the Life of every living thing, He governs all things in perpetual goodness and incorruptible perfection...for that is the nature of His Life. In others words, I begin to realize Omnipresence and Omnipotence! As I allow myself to flow into Omnipotence I embrace whatever the situation, and all those involved, into this space of God "all in all." He then becomes *the only governing influence and always for good, always for perfection and harmony and restoration.*

In accepting God as the Life, as the Presence and the Power, I have accepted Him also as the Wisdom...no longer trying to impose my own thoughts and ways upon the situation. I have in essence, "died to self." I have proved my trust and therefore my love.

After experiencing this for quite sometime and consistently seeing the effect upon the human scene, I began to feel that this Life is also Love. Soon Love itself began to permeate the atmosphere and space it lived in. I felt the Love of the Earth. No longer simply as ball of stone to walk upon and feed from. But as a living, giving, loving, created being...and in doing so, I fell in love with Love. I wanted to respect this Earth in that it had become Love itself to me. It gave and gave, faithfully and predictably and we took and took. Now I wanted to love and care for it in return. Again fulfilling the saying, "If you choose to live unto yourself, you shall lose your life, but if you give (casting your bread upon the waters of life) you shall surely gain your life."

As I continued on this path I was soon able to feel the Life and Love of all mankind. It was then easy to see beyond the human insanity and confusion and fear. I felt the Life and I felt the Love. It was all God, all good, all perfect...for He is altogether good and perfect. That Life became once again Omnipotent, ruling over and swallowing up all evil imaginations appearing as disease, despair, depression, all human misery. I realized I was not loving the Lord, my God with all my heart, soul, mind and strength unless I was seeing Him as the Life of it all and blessing that Life.

Do not confuse morality with spirituality. Morality does not produce spirituality. But true spirituality will produce morality. So we will never progress in our unfoldment as the mighty and loving Sons of God by being good, or maintaining human standards of behavior. But only by entering into the Life that is above, beneath, within and without all things. And loving it...for it is Love.

We release ownership of all things and in doing so find we possess the fullness of Him who sent us, filled us and loves us. Our bodies are not our possessions. Our careers are not our possessions. Our money is not our possession, our relationship are not to be personally possessed. Our children are not ours to possess. Our homes, our properties, our everything and anything is not ours...but simply manifestations of that Life and declarations of that Love. He who formed all this is the Life of it and is more than able to maintain it in perpetual Divine Order. For His nature is immutable (unchangeable,) indestructible, incorruptible and perfect.

"For when this mortal shall have put on immortality and this corruptible shall have put on incorruptibility, then we shall all be changed and death shall be swallowed up by Life."

CHAPTER SIXTEEN

CAST YOUR BREAD
UPON THE WATERS

"Cast your bread upon the waters...for you shall find it after many days." (Ecclesiastes 11:1)

How are we to live now that we know who we are? How does the Son of God, the Light unto the world live?

Living out from the Christ consciousness is *living to give*...unlike the human consciousness which is forever chasing after what one can *get*. To live to give is the way to Life.

Dis-ease... whether of the mind, the body, the home, the finances, the relationships, whatever...is always a result of a choking down of the Life giving Spirit of Life within.

We choke down when our focus is to get, to add to, instead of give out. To preserve our substance, we hold onto our means. To preserve our relationships we maintain a certain amount of control. To preserve our position we seek to protect our jobs from another moving into our place. We seek to protect our interests from competitors. We seek to hold onto and protect everything we hold dear to us for fear that we will lose. We live out from a thought that there is a limited supply of whatever and we must hold onto our share of it or be without!

We don't see this Divine Life in which "we live and move and have our being" as the source of all we have…and therefore *unable to be limited.* We don't understand that to give, to pour out from within our being, is to *make room for more to enter*!

There are so many ways to express this Life but none so profound as to give. To give is always to receive a greater measure than we gave. A clenched fist cannot receive anything, but an open hand can hold much.

As we allow this Life force to be poured out from the midst of our souls, it flows through our being from the True Source, through us and back to the True Source again. While this Life is flowing it is demonstrating its nature to and through us. This is when healings happen!

"For of Him and through him and to Him are all things." It must be an uninterrupted circle of unobstructed flow in order to realize the Greatness and abundance of the Spirit of God.

It manifests as strength to and through our bodies, a sense of wholeness and contentment to our minds. It demonstrates as Wisdom and direction, council and understanding. It demonstrates as friendship, trusting companionship, mutual respect, joyful interactions. It demonstrates as wholeness and harmony in the body, the workplace, the home, everywhere we live. It causes us to see beauty all around us and to feel apart of the Life of all things.

To give is to live.

If our purse, our salary, our banker, our investments are the source of our money, we will have a sense of limitation. But if this Life, which is Eternal God, is the never-ending source, we will feel free to pour out to others freely. As we give from our supply, we find ourselves receiving beyond what we imagined we ever needed.

If we see God as the Life of others, we will trust, we will love unhesitantly, we will look beyond faults and human frailties. We will give love freely. We will forgive quickly and often. As we forgive others, we will find Mercy and tenderness when we ourselves fail. We will never be afraid to ask for forgiveness, because we will trust the hearts of others, knowing they possess the heart of God. We will never hold onto pride... clinging to it, wrapping it about our hearts as a shawl... as though it were protecting our very life, when in fact it is the source of death. Instead we will humbly give and receive forgiveness and Love.

We will be confident in the Wisdom and decisions we entertain and share, because we know the Source of all Wisdom and understanding is the One Mind which we possess. We will pause and ask the Spirit of Counsel and Direction, and then move forward with assurance that the Spirit goes before us.

As we pour out happiness, joyfulness, hope and encouragement, we will find ourselves enjoying these thoughts in our own lives. A simple compliment coming from a sincere heart, a smile of encouragement, a gentle touch will restore a heart lost in a sense of isolation.

We heal others by simple acts of tenderness, mercy and forgiveness. As we do this for others, we are able to receive it for ourselves when needed.

"Greater love than this hath no man, but that he lay down his life for another." This is how we are to lay down our lives. Give...pour out from your substance. Laugh, love and live. Only judgments, criticisms, opinions, and haughty attitudes will block this. If someone is behaving in a destructive manner to themselves or another, your criticism will not heal them. But your Love and Mercy and forgiveness will.

Disease cannot remain. Poverty cannot remain. Loneliness cannot remain. Fractured relationships cannot remain. *These are not things that need to be healed, as people think!* These are obstructions to the flow of Life that need to be *removed.* To open the heart and to give is to remove these obstructions.

To give is to live.

CHAPTER SEVENTEEN

TEACH US TO PRAY

Without a doubt this is the most repeated question I have heard throughout my life. "How should I pray about this?" "Am I praying wrong that this has not resolved?" "Is there some other way that I should be praying that I haven't found yet?"

As long as I live I will never forget the pleading in my sister's voice when she asked me this question. My heart died within me because I knew she had in her mind a God who must be approached in some perfect manner or she would not be heard. She saw God as a separate Being from her and far, far away... difficult to be entreated. She saw herself as needing to overcome God's "reluctance" to help her by some magic prayer. How many hearts are also filled with such a distorted image of God? How many hearts fail in despair because of this common belief presented to us for centuries by those who supposedly represented God to us? How wonderful beyond description will it be when mankind is so familiarized with the truth of God that we never hear this again? For when we know Him as He truly is, "we *shall be like Him*, for we will see Him *as He is*." "The earth shall be filled with the knowledge of the Lord as the waters cover the sea." "And no man shall have to say to his neighbor, 'Know the Lord,' for all shall know me from the least to the greatest." When we *know* Him, not just know *about* Him, prayer is so comfortable, so natural, so easy and so confident, we will never hear such pleading and despair again. "Acquaint yourself with him and be at peace, thereby your good shall come to you."

There are several things that need to be known or re-membered here.

First is that God is not a God who loves, but is Love, Itself. God is not a God who shows mercy to some and not to others less worthy. God Is Mercy, Itself. He cannot go against His own nature. "He cannot deny Himself."

A long time ago I had a discussion with a woman who was "in the ministry." I told her that I had been stopped on the highway for speeding but that I had prayed for mercy and the officer only gave me a warning ticket instead. She was incensed! She said since I was speeding and I deserved a ticket, I had no business asking for mercy. I deserved to be punished! Well, while I couldn't deny that I deserved to be punished, I knew that God was Mercy and Mercy would cover my offense because I asked for it. It would lift me above the punishment due. What is Mercy anyway except choosing to forgive offenses and deal in goodness instead of punishment? *God deals with us according to HIS OWN heart and nature...not according to our offenses*! She obviously had never knowingly received mercy nor had she knowingly offered anyone mercy. She was trying to win God's favor by doing good...but who does good always? Not me! And is there such a phenomena as "God's favor?" God is Love and only Love. "Favor" or anything needing to be earned is not Love at all.

The new covenant, or promise, which God revealed to His Creation by Jesus, was that He would *cover* mankind with His Spirit and *cause* them to live in righteousness... again by His Spirit. He said "Their sins and iniquities (He) would remember no more." This is Mercy, that God would do for us what we could not do for ourselves.

Mankind lived under the law of sowing and reaping, cause and effect... and that new terminology now, the law of attraction... for generations, until Jesus. "The law came by Moses, but Mercy and truth came by Jesus Christ.

"We have not because we ask not." We all need Mercy. We all offend. To approach God knowing that He is Mercy and delights in our receiving it, is to know God! To approach God expecting punishment, knowing we deserve it, is a declaration that we don't know Him at all!

The whole religious world is so afraid that if we talk about Mercy, man will continue to sin. Well we've talked about punishment for centuries and that has not deterred mankind from sinning yet! No, "Mercy rejoices against judgment!" If you have ever received Mercy when you knew that you deserved to be punished, you have just stood face to face with God Himself. You would never be the same again and you would learn to show Mercy to others you encounter.

So, when you approach God, know that you are approaching Mercy and expect that you will receive it. This blesses the heart of God as in no other way. If you have offended… if you think you said or did or believed in a way that drew this into your experience… then immediately repent. Choose again. Reject it from your soul. Send it away. That is all it takes… and it must go…along with all the punishment deserved by it. Once you have done that, move on. There is no need to do it again in this situation. If there is someone you have injured by offense or by omission, quickly repent and begin to pray in earnest for that person, whether they are alive or have gone on. If you feel that you should speak to that person, ask God for Wisdom and His timing. He will direct when Wisdom deems it right to approach the one offended.

Forgive and you shall be forgiven! Then Mercy can flow.

The second thing that needs to be remembered when you pray is that God is never reluctant to help. You don't ever need to think that you must overcome God's reluctance to help… for two reasons. One is that it is the Eternal purpose and Divine Intention throughout Eternity *for Life to be revealed*. God is Life, the Life of you and all Creation. He flows through Creation as an unseen, uninterruptible force of beauty and harmony. It is His intention that His Life be expressed, revealed and fully manifested. We must not wait for the circumstances to be perfect to claim the Perfection of Life.

So healing and restoration of all situations and circumstances is always the will and intention of God. Never, never, does He use evil to gain good. He uses Mercy to gain good. God does not use evil for anything. Evil is not an entity to be used or not used, but it is simply the absence of Goodness experienced. When Goodness is not being consciously realized, evil can move into that space in soul. It is darkness. When light moves in darkness flees. When goodness, and expectation of goodness moves in, evil appearances vanish. Your suffering is not from God and has absolutely no good reason to exist or to continue.

God wants His Life, which is your Life, to be revealed...that will be healing. That will be goodness, harmony, abundance, contentment and peace. That will be "As it is in heaven, so shall it be in earth." All the promises of God are "Yea and amen!" God is always saying yes!

Another thing worthy to consider when approaching God in prayer is that nothing new needs to be created here. Nothing new added. Nothing new at all. Only something, the Life of God, needs to be seen, expressed. It comes up from deep inside your soul and *is your very soul*. It will surface and when it does you will say you have been healed. But really your real and Eternal nature has been revealed. God isn't taking something sick and making it well. The Life of God is never sick. God isn't taking something poor and making it prosperous. God isn't taking something evil and making it good. God isn't taking something lacking and making it enriched and whole. You are whole and complete as you stand right now. God is simply revealing what already is and always will be. Nothing new needs to be created. All the creating that needed to be done was done a long, long time ago. So we *let* God appear. We bless this Life that resides within us and we let it appear. It wants to!

ᚼ THE LORD'S
PRAYER

We read in the 11th chapter of Luke where the followers of Jesus asked him to teach them how to pray.

Prayer is progressive in nature. We pray according to our understanding of God. Unfortunately if we are still locked in the traditional image of God, that distortion leads us to think of God as one who is separate and apart from us. One who may have a good reason for our suffering and just might not want to relieve us.

But if we have progressed beyond that evil imagination of God, we at least know that all the promises of God are, "Yea, and Amen!" God always says "Yes!" We shouldn't outline *how* the prayer is to be answered, but only to have the utmost confidence that it will be *wonderful beyond imagination*. "Exceedingly abundantly above all that we could ask or think."

Later we may be at the place in understanding that it is accepting the *thoughts and beliefs* of mass, unenlightened world consciousness, which is causing what we are experiencing, for good or evil. Jesus said, "According to your (beliefs, faith, understanding)...so shall it be done unto you." Unfortunately our beliefs often are quite different than what we wish we could experience. We want to experience something different, but deep down inside we still believe that there is a power of evil that will win. It is those beliefs which need to be corrected. And we do this by bringing in a higher, more truthful and Eternal belief system...replacing the one we have been taught all our lives. When we understand that "As a man thinketh in his heart, so is he," it is no wonder at all that we suffer with unimaginable diseases and miseries. We believe that misery is the prevailing experience in this life and that God has so ordained it. Until we radically extricate our souls from such death producing hysteria, we shall continue to suffer.

Our only prayer should be to line up with the Eternal Mind of God...for all He knows is goodness and perfection. That is the immutable, (unchangeable) uninterrupted, incorruptible, indestructible, absolute, Eternal truth. God sees what God has made. And "all the works of His hands are perfect." No matter what we are seeing right now, no matter how long it has prevailed, no matter how many doctors have told us that there is no hope, no matter how many people have believed that... and died right on schedule...in the Mind that is God, all that exists is Present Perfection. It is always our distorted image of things that needs to be corrected. So we are not asking God to change anything at all. Only to enable us, who already "have the mind of Christ," to realize what is already perfect, whole and complete. As our perception changes, as our beliefs change, our experience will change with no effort at all on the human plane.

There is really no wrong way to pray. Just as my grandson, now 2 years old, speaks to me in a way that is typical of his development, I hear and I understand and I respond. I love him and of course I will respond however he communicates with me. And so it is with God. We are so loved, so cherished, so cared for, that no matter how we talk to God...so long as we speak from our hearts and not from a book with no real feeling involved... we shall be heard. Every prayer I have ever uttered to God has been answered. I expect that it will, just as my grandson knows that I will respond to him.

When the disciples asked Jesus to teach them how to pray, he of course responded with what we all refer to as The Lord's prayer, but we stop short of all that he taught us here. First of all I now believe that the prayer was really teaching us about God so that we could know the Nature of Him to Whom we pray. I'm not so sure that we were simply to repeat it, although there is power in those words, as there are in all the words of Jesus, for he spoke the words of God.

Let's first break down that prayer and then go on with the remainder of his teaching on the subject.

"Our Father which art in heaven..."

God is the source and origin of us all, saint and sinner alike. We don't one day become His offspring. We have always been so from before the foundation of the world. In the body or out of the body, we are created by and come *out from* Him. Heaven is the place and space where pure understanding supplants the error we have all experienced. It is within us all and without. It fills all space even though we don't necessarily see that. It is here and now, for Jesus said that the "Kingdom of God is within you." That means that we possess all the dominion, authority, power and strength which is found in the Kingdom. A kingdom is a place where there is one authority and one absolute power. It is the power of the king. And we are called, "kings and priests, unto God."

He told us all to "Go, preach that the Kingdom of Heaven is here." He declared that was his real mission. To place heaven back into the hearts of men and out from the sky, far, far away. He never said we could only enter it when we died. He never said that we couldn't experience it till we died. Not physically died anyway. He never said that we needed to "earn" our way there either! Only "repent" to enter in. Only choose another way, another thought, another belief. Only let go of all that holds us to the old thinking. Only release our souls from the prison of strange, insane doctrines of men. When we have become willing to do that, we simply enter in. This is the real "death to self" that we must experience in order to find ourselves immersed in the Eternal Heaven of the soul.

"Hallowed be thy name."

I always consciously move into the Presence of God by remembering the wonderful Nature and attributes of God. I recall His power, His dominion, His Love and Life. I acknowledge that He fills all space and He is perfect and glorious in His Being. God doesn't need all this exaltation. I do. I need to remind myself that all I have been seeing in the world is not the truth about God. I need to remember that He is the *all and only* power, and that power is only good. I need this to shake off the madness of "world thought" that might be clinging to my soul so that I can enter His Presence with confidence and wonder. I can then expect only goodness. I am assured that His purpose and intention in all His dealings with man is to bring forth His Life, through us, and to us, and for us.

So we exalt the "Name of the Lord." Since God lives in our soul, deep within our being... as we lift up His Name, His Nature...we can feel ourselves becoming stronger and more confident. It can literally be felt as we speak. Many times that is all it takes to deliver us from the most obtrusive experiences and conditions. It would be good to spend an hour or so remembering and speaking and perhaps even writing, all that we know about the goodness and Glory of God. Psalm 37 says, we must "delight ourselves in the Lord and He will give us the desires of our hearts."

"Thy Kingdom come, Thy will be done, on Earth as it is in Heaven."

The will of God is always that all the beauty and order and perfection of Heaven be established right here, right now. He wants to release Heaven from within our souls, out into visible manifestation. This is how the Kingdom is to come and appear "on Earth as in Heaven." From within our being...outwards.

This will translate into health, order, harmony, balance, love, respect, honor, abundance, tenderness and goodness... radiant Glory. It is no wonder then that we really don't need to outline our wants and desires..."For your Father knows you have need of all these things." Everything we can possibly need is included in the coming of this Kingdom. Or, better put, in the revealing of the Life of God from within our very souls.

"Give us this day our daily bread."

If we think that our supply comes from our bank account, our job, our resources, we are walking precariously on the edge of a precipice. If we think that way, what happens to us when the job fails, the money dries up, the human source changes? What happens when we can't work anymore, when we are doing all that we are capable of and it ceases to be sufficient for our needs? When human resources fail, we must learn this truth. God is the supply of all our needs. What we need appears...period. Actually the only thing that can possibly block this is when we have our own "ways and means" in the way. *Human effort is the single greatest enemy of our goodness appearing.* When we can't or won't let go and let God supply for us. It is the evidence that we don't believe. That we don't trust. Pray to trust. Pray for a trusting heart. This is true for every need.

"And forgive us our trespasses (sins) as we forgive others their trespasses."

This is so critical to any healing that I have reserved a separate chapter for this topic alone. "As" is the operative word here. *As* we allow Mercy and grace to pour out from us, *as* we live in Love and allow Love to pour out from us...even in our thoughts...especially in our thoughts!...we will also be released from whatever blocks or stands in the way of the flow of Life or healing that *we* need.

"Lead us not into temptation, but deliver us from evil."

Do not allow us to be led into evil. James says that we are drawn away into temptation by our own thoughts. God couldn't lead us into evil. It would be contrary to His entire Nature to do so and there would be no reason to do so.

But let's talk about temptation here for a minute. Temptation is what it's all about. It's not about a disease appearing. It's not about anything appearing in the material world. Everything begins with a thought. We can reject the thought or accept the thought as valid and real and powerful. So, for instance, if we are facing a disease process, it began with a temptation, a thought. It's says something like this. "I am more powerful than God. I have the capacity to destroy this body, this mind. I have done this to many in the past and no one has ever been able to stop me. I am death and I am more powerful than Life."

But God says this. "I am the all and only power. I am the Life of every living thing. I am the substance of every living thing. Nothing can... or ever has... or ever will interrupt this. You, my beloved, have believed more in the temptation, the thought that is contrary to this, than you have to this truth. Therefore you have experienced suffering. But you can repent of this right now. You can be released from this and all the effects of this right now. You can be filled with grace right now and you then will believe that "I am He and there is no other!" Don't believe your eyes. Don't believe your ears either. Don't believe what you may be feeling. Whatever is contrary to this absolute truth is not truth at all, but only a mass, hypnotic belief that has enslaved the people since the beginning of time. You can break out of this. You must break out of this. We do this not by our own efforts, but *by grace*. By the workings of the Spirit of God within us. This Spirit is released as soon as we make the way clear for it to flow and we do this by a simple act of repentance. "I choose to release my soul from this belief. I choose the Mind, that is God, to fill my space, my very existence right now." "For it is not by might (human), not by power (human), but by my Spirit, says the Lord. This mountain shall be removed, *by my Spirit.*"

This is all it takes and soon our heart is less fearful. Soon our mind is more relaxed. Soon we are calm and peaceful and we begin to feel confidence and quietness and assurance. Soon we actually are experiencing what God knows eternally as truth.

Now we must stay with this day and night until the work is completed. The thought, the temptation to be drawn back into the insanity is always lurking about "seeking whom it may devour." Don't let it be you. It takes perseverance, but the result is worth the insistence on the truth. Anything of any consequence takes practice and focus. This is why we are referred to as disciples. It takes discipline!

ಌ PERSISTENCE
IN PRAYER

Now we might think that the instruction to the disciples is finished here, but not so!

He goes on to tell a story about a man who went to his neighbor's house very late one night asking for bread to give to an unexpected guest that arrived at his house, as he was without sufficient food to serve this guest. The neighbor at first refused because his whole household was already asleep for the night, but when he saw that this man was not going to leave without the desired bread, he finally gave in and fulfilled the request.

Years ago this story bothered me. It made me image a God who needed to be begged for what we needed. So I begged a lot and I received a lot. It was much later that I realized that it is *impossible for Divine Love to withhold anything at any time for any reason*. I realized that it is *for our benefit* that we need to remain persistent. There are so many layers of unbelief and false ideology that need to be removed for us to receive and this is the way to remove them. With each approach to God in prayer, the layers are peeled back and we finally are at a position to experience what has been available to us all along.

He goes on to tell us to "ask and keep on asking." "To seek and keep on seeking"…never letting go until we have what we need. He says for us to knock and the door to our soul, where all the goodness of God resides, will be opened to us.

Every prayer will be answered. Every request for help will be given.

This reminds me of the story of Jacob and Esau, two twin brothers who had a serious falling out and separated for many years. But Esau's hate and grudge remained and years later Jacob was about to face his brother, who he had deliberately and deeply offended and he feared for his life. All night long before this meeting was to take place, Jacob remained in prayer. At one point, while he "wrestled with the angel" sent to minister to him, the angel was about to leave him and he took hold of the angel and refused to let him go. He said, "I will not let you go till you bless me!" This is the level of insistence that we need to open the doors of the soul when we have shut down the flow of Divine Life. It helps us to define our intention and desire and frees us to receive the solution. In this case when he saw his brother, Esau, it says, "He saw as it were the face of God." At that point the brothers were able to reconcile and peace was restored.

It has been long established that the point at which we can truly "see" the Christ within another, we are healed. For this is the true and everlasting essence of who we all are. This is the "establishment of the Kingdom of God on earth."

It was Jacob's unwillingness to "let go," even when it looked like the help was not going to appear, that brought victory to the situation.

Continuing on in Luke we read where Jesus defines the Nature of God to us so that we can *expect* goodness to appear. It is this clear definition of the unchangeable nature of Divine Love which silences the mouths of all unbelief and fear. "Which of you will give to your own children a serpent, when he asks you for a fish to eat? Which of you will give a stone to your children when he asks of you a piece of bread to eat? Or if he asks for an egg will you give him a scorpion instead? If you know how to give good gifts to your own children, how much more shall your Heavenly Father give (The Holy Spirit) to him that asks?"

I love this portion of scripture. It settles once and for all the intention and purpose of God to always care for us and to help us in time of need. This… forever in my mind… buries the awful religious image of a god who sends sickness and defeat "for our own good, or that good may appear!" This reveals the "heart of Love" and ought to give us the peace we need and the confidence in Love's care for us, to rise above any situation with victory.

Notice also that He says, "…will He give the *Holy Spirit* to him that asks…" He is declaring to us that contained within this Spirit of Eternal Life, the same Spirit that motivated Jesus to do and accomplish all that he did, is all that could ever be needed for any and all situations we will ever wrestle with here in this human condition. I remember the day, long, long ago when it suddenly came to me, "If I had the Spirit flowing right now, that is really all I would ever need!" And it has been ever since!

I am not going to outline a specific way to pray, no more than I would tell someone how to talk with a best friend, or a lover. I will say that the more relaxed and intimate you are with God, the better able you will be to hear Him when He answers you. I also will warn you against any formality in prayer.

Many pray using affirmations of what is always true and never can be altered. Many, myself included, use Scripture references that really speak to my heart…words that cannot be altered. These are prayers acknowledging truth and being grateful for the immutability of the truth. This is a wonderful tool to enable you to enter a peaceful state in order to hear the word of God. If you are still wandering around in the wilderness of confusion and very affected by whatever is disturbing you, just talk with God and be at peace with that. The words of truth are imperative, but without the Spirit of truth, they become empty words. Just speak with God and grace will soon fill your heart and those words will become Life to you and healing to the situation.

"If you abide in me, and my words *abide in you*, you shall ask what you will and it *shall be done unto you.*" Walk with Him, talk with Him. The more aggressive the appearance of the evil, the more you will want to separate yourself from others and be with Him. Abide with Him and soon you will be abiding *in* Him. It is then that you will truly know your absolute "oneness" with your Creator.

"...Whatsoever you shall ask the Father *in my name,* He will do it for you." "In his name" is being in the same Spirit and thought that resided in Jesus.

One such thought that resided in the heart of Jesus would be a full realization that we have come to *serve a purpose greater than our own*...a desire to be a vehicle of expression of the Nature of God, to, in and through us.

The opposite of this intention is to attempt to use the Principles of Truth to serve our own selfish and self serving wants, which unfortunately is a thought which is running rampant among many churches these days. But we are persuaded of a better way. We have come to "serve a purpose greater than our own!"

CHAPTER EIGHTEEN

TO HEAR THE WORD OF GOD

"The ear of the wise seeketh knowledge."

Proverbs 18:15

"He waketh my ear to hear." Is. 50:4

When we are in trouble we concern ourselves with whether or not God is hearing our cry for help. He says, "Before you called I heard and while you were yet speaking, I answered." We are always being heard. Saint and sinner alike, God hears the cry of every creature created. "He opens His hand and satisfies the desire of every living thing."

The real concern here should not be so much, "Is God hearing me?" But the real issue is. "Are we hearing God?" Because when we do hear the Word that He speaks, we will be healed! "He sent His Word and it healed them." And so it is. When we are able to hear His Word concerning any situation at all, the darkness is swallowed up by the sheer power of His Word. This is one of those "across the board" absolutes. When God speaks the issue is resolved.

Previously we spoke about the intention of God is always to reveal His Life in every situation. So we can safely rest in the assurance that God is always moving in the direction of revealing Life where death, disease, despair and darkness of any form is present. We should settle this once and for all in our hearts. God never uses evil that good may come. God is the Ever Present Goodness and certainly doesn't need evil to help Him to appear. It is not suffering that causes evil to vanish and goodness to appear. It is His Word that causes goodness to appear. When He speaks, the earth melts and the clouds disappear.

Can we hear the Voice of God? Not only *can* we, but multitudes of times we are *instructed* to hear His Voice in order to live. It is not a matter of "getting God to speak" but of hearing what He is already saying. There are many ways that God communicates with His beloved man and He alone knows the way that will reach our heart in any given situation. So we leave the "how to" to Divine Wisdom and just rest, knowing that He will speak in a way each one of us can hear best. When our infant children needed to realize our love, we spoke in a way that was different than we did to our toddler children, who also needed to realize our love and perhaps our instructions as well. This again will be different as we approach adulthood and so on. God is Wisdom Itself and knows what we need in order to realize His will, His intention, His mind on any matter. This will be our healing..

Do we need to qualify in order to hear? In a way, yes! If we are afraid of what we might hear, we will unconsciously shut out the hearing. If we are afraid, that is a sure declaration that we don't know the reality of the Nature of God as Love. This is understandable since we have all been instructed in various religions as well as the general world thought about the nature and ways of God, which is distorted and an "evil imagination" of God. If this is our problem the solution is simple. We must just *ask God* to show us who He really is and prove to us that He will always lead us in a way that will secure goodness to us. It may not be exactly as you are demanding, but if not, it will be better! He says, "Taste of me and prove me and see if there be any wicked way in me." "Prove me and see that I am good."

So God understands the horror we have been fed all these generations concerning Him and He is ready and desirous to correct such a convoluted and evil image.

The second way we "qualify" is that we must be willing to obey His Voice, which is easy to do when we realize Him as the loving Shepherd of our soul and our Life. "My sheep hear my voice and no other voice will they follow." This is the heart that leaves the 99 sheep to find the one that is lost. If that is you or the one you are praying for, be at peace! He will not rest until He holds that one in His loving arms!

So the second easily follows the first. Just ask Him to fix your heart. And He will. Tell Him if you are afraid of Him and find it hard to trust Him. And ask for that to be replaced with understanding and confidence. And He will.

We all have to sooner or later leave the idea of "us trying to hold onto God," and replace it with the realization that God is holding onto us! "Fear not, little flock. It is your Father's good pleasure to give you His kingdom." Such is the essence of Divine Love.

God sends His Spirit to go before us in every situation in order to "make the crooked ways straight." When we learn this and begin to live by it our lives become peaceful and confident and restful. We begin to feel loved and cherished and in a continual state of care and protection. We realize we are being guided into greater wonders of Love and we cease to fear or doubt. When situations arise, we simply pause with an expectation that we will know the direction we are to go. This will be the solution to the issue, no matter what it may be. "And you shall hear a word behind you saying, 'This is the way, walk in it!'"

The whole book of Proverbs tells us the value of allowing Divine Wisdom to rule all our affairs. It says that health, prosperity, long life, honor and goodness will be the measure of our expectation if we let Wisdom govern.

James says that if we ask for Wisdom, it will appear to us. But he cautions us to be clear that God will indeed answer us and not to doubt. Doubting is a habit just like worrying is a habit. We can stop all that with just making a choice to trust. "I choose to trust. I choose to follow the guidance of Spirit in this situation. I choose to hear direction clearly. I choose to trust." Saying this often throughout the day will settle our heart and bring us a measure of peace which will allow us to hear and to know. We must repent of the doubts. Just release them by an act of our choice, our will. They will go. And choose again. This time choose to trust. *When we do this we are reprogramming our expectations and therefore our experiences.*

I have never known a person who wanted to learn to "hear" the voice of Wisdom and have not heard it. The desire to do so is the only prerequisite. Spend as much time alone as possible. Go for walks alone, without the cell phone or head phones. Learn to enjoy the quietness and peace. The world is afraid of quietness and peace. It terrifies them because it begins to move them towards the things of Eternity. But that is exactly what we are longing for, so again, choose again. Choose times of aloneness and you will find that you seek it more and more. For it is then that you are renewed and refreshed and guided into confidence and assurance, strength and power.

"In the day that you seek me with your whole heart, I will be found of you." (Jeremiah 29:13) "Call unto me and I will answer you and show you great and mighty things which you knew not." (Jeremiah 33:3)

CHAPTER NINETEEN

GUARD YOUR WORDS

"By your words you are either justified or condemned!"
Jesus...Matthew

"The issues of life and death are in the power of the tongue!"
Proverbs

Often folks consider that this must mean we *create* the tragedies we experience, or the good that we experience, by what we speak. We don't. Really it means that we demonstrate what we *actually believe is true* by what we speak. It may not be what we *wished* we believed or what we wanted to see happen, but our words do tell us what we are holding deep within our hearts as the truth for us. The good thing about that is that when we hear ourselves speak, and know that it came from the belief system deep in our hearts, it gives us a place to start in our healing. It actually tells us what *belief* needs to be healed for the physical appearance, for the life issue, to be corrected.

So we read, "Out from the abundance of the heart the mouth speaks." You cannot be holding in your heart one belief, say, in the power of "this disease," and then think that by saying something different you will cause what you desire to appear. It doesn't work that way. You must maintain silence "before the Lord" until the necessary change happens *in your heart*.

And how does this happen? Ask God to change your heart. Repent of the power you have given to this situation or this condition. It is no power at all, but a *belief* in a power. Repent for believing that something in all of God's Creation can have the power to usurp authority over God Himself, over Eternal Life, Itself. Then ask God to free you of this belief and to replace it with His Mind...that which is, and always has been, Eternally true.
Then wait.

Whenever the fear or worry or fretting returns, repent again...and ask again. Stay with it until the change comes. It will, I promise. Don't discuss this with anyone. This is between you and God. This is going on in your soul and not in the courthouse of public opinions and conclusions.

Thought is energy. By thought and intention you are deliberately releasing energy where you are placing your focus.

When you have been filled with the thought contained within Divine Mind, you are sensing the Life force or Spirit. You are becoming aware of it and by doing so you are releasing it and exalting it, magnifying it...increasing its intensity within your soul.

All modalities will only give temporary relief from suffering. This is because they deal on a superficial level, not addressing the consciousness or belief of the individual, which is where the problems originate. It is only by a change of consciousness that the desired change will be permanent. This is not accomplished by trying to convince anyone of truth or by them trying to convince themselves. It is done solely by grace. It is done on a spiritual level by the effectual workings of the Holy Spirit and not on a mental level at all. While we may start on a mental level by declaring what we realize is the unchangeable Eternal truth, (it is true that a working understanding of the absolute truth of the Present Perfection of man, created in the image of his maker, is necessary and to be desired,) it is not by this intellectual mental understanding that a permanent change will be achieved.

An understanding of the true Nature of God and the Eternal intention of His heart to reveal His Life in every situation offered to Him is a wonderful place to rest your heart. To know that God *always* wants, and is intent on revealing, absolute wholeness and goodness and the abundance of all Life, for that is who He is…is undeniably the single greatest revelation we can receive. But even that will not make a change in the human condition *until the Spirit of God is allowed to flow. Until grace is the working energy and not man's efforts.* When it is flowing even infants and children can easily benefit, although unable to understand the hidden mysteries of the Love that is God.

169

Your words are the most powerful energy given to man. It is your sword of authority, your power and your dominion. By your word heaven appears in hell. But your word is nothing unless it is the word that you have "heard" in the silence with God. Jesus said that "As (he) heard, so he did." He said that (he) "could of his own self do nothing," but solely depended upon following whatever the Spirit spoke to his heart. He learned to depend upon that "word" for everything he did and to know that with absolute assurance what he spoke would come to pass...because he heard it. So we read, "Faith cometh by hearing and hearing by the word of God."

Now, how do we get to the hearing phase? "You have not because you ask not." You will begin to hear simply by asking to hear. Simply by desiring to know what is the Mind and heart of God on any particular subject.

I always begin by remembering and declaring that I possess the Mind of God. That the Mind of God and I are One in substance and One in being. I cannot therefore be separated from what God knows or from what God is declaring. I always begin by asking to have the thoughts of God revealed to me so that I will pray according to the will and purpose of God. Then I *know* the healing or correction will appear.

First we must realize that God wants to, and is, communicating with man from the time we were sent here. This goes on no matter who we are or how we have lived our life. But it takes a commitment to the purposes of God, a surrender to His ways in order to hear. Just as the radio station is always broadcasting, God is always revealing his intentions to man. But again, just like the radio, we must tune in. We must learn to be in touch with the frequency. There is a vibration, so to speak, that is unique to God alone. It is the vibration of Wisdom. James says that if you ask for Wisdom, Wisdom will come.

Although many subscribe to long periods of silence and meditation to hear from God, I never have. I find that the effort of silencing my own mind blocks out the easy vibration and impulse of Spirit. I love to read my Bible. I love to read the writings of those who have "walked the walk and not just talked the talk." I love to take walks with God and just visit with Him about my day, my patients, what I should know and what I should do in any given situation. I do this all the time, whether awake, working, driving, doing my chores at home or visiting with patients at the clinic. I do this in my sleep I think because I hear a lot from God during those night time hours. I never try to generate it. I never try to interfere at all. I want to hear a pure word and not the foolishness and chatter from my own mind. "Blessed be God who reveals His thoughts to man."

This is best accomplished by not having a "vested interest" in the outcome. "Commit your ways unto the Lord and your thoughts shall be established." I know it is beyond me to force, or even to necessarily know, how God will appear...how the healing or restoration will come. It is enough for me to know that He will. And when He does, Heaven appears. All the authority, dominion, strength, Wisdom, might and Majesty appears and darkness just vanishes away into its native state of nothingness. The heart and mind is completely captured by this experience and all is well. Whether I see it or not right away is immaterial to me. I am filled with contentment and joy anyway and I know it will appear. And it always has and it always will. And for you too! Often times "exceedingly abundantly above all that we could ask or think."

King David never made a move without consulting Divine Wisdom, even if the answer seemed obvious to him. Therefore God called him "a man after his own heart." A man who sought after the heart and Mind of God. Therefore he was exalted far above all other kings and men. Therefore he always succeeded in all the situations that he faced.

Now his predecessor, Saul, failed to establish the kingdom simply because he failed to ask, to wait, to hear and to obey what he heard. Because of this lack of surrender and apparent self-will, the kingdom crashed and was taken into captivity by their enemies. Had he sincerely repented, the whole mess would have been washed away and success would have followed. But he never did.

We must use Wisdom as to what we allow to enter our minds, our atmospheres of thought. We must flee from empty talking. It is not only a waste of time, a distraction from "hearing," but "In the multitude of words there is always sin."

Meaning that we are bound to say or agree with something which is not the absolute pure, present perfection of God and man, in His image. We are bound to confess something which we don't want to experience...forgetting that we establish our experiences by our words, "for out of the abundance of the heart, the mouth speaks."

It was said of Samuel that God "let none of his words fall to the ground." Every word he spoke had an effect. And so it is with us, though we are sometimes far from being convinced of this.

The more we make a conscious effort to watch our words the more we will realize just how often we say things that are less than the uninterrupted truth and something we would not wish to experience. This is a good time for us to pray for the grace to guard our thoughts and our words.

"Let your words be few. Even a fool is counted wise when he holds his tongue."

Wait in the silence of your soul till the Word of God is formed in your mind. Then speak that Word and the healing will follow. The power of your words in this capacity will astound you. Do not be discouraged by the length of time it might take. Sometimes it is immediate and sometimes it is days, even weeks ...but always it will come. And it will be the power of God unto the situation.

Father, as I wait upon you my memory strays to the innumerable times I have allowed nonsense to fill my mind and been entertained by the insanities of the world. The thousands of words we have foolishly and idly spoken. And for all this we repent. We reject it all from our souls. As we take hold of Mercy and grace and realize we are washed clean, a space is provided...as space of anticipation is cre-

ated. All sin is removed. A space is created for you, for Spirit, for your word of Wisdom. Your word, your truth, your intention and purposes are invited to be spoken and realized now. I wait with confidence. I wait with anticipation. For your word is my freedom and my power.

GUARD YOUR THOUGHTS

Without the discipline of "bringing every thought into captivity to the truth of Christ" preeminent in your life, you will inadvertently allow any thought that's swarms about your mind to enter in and find a home. Every thought you entertain will find some form of expression in your life. For good or ill, we live out from what we have put into our minds. Therefore we are instructed in 11Corinthians 10:5..."Casting down imaginations, and every high thing that exhalteth itself against the knowledge of God, and bringing every thought to obedience of Christ..."

If thoughts, words, beliefs, concepts and ideologies could be seen or measured we would be amazed to find that we live in an atmosphere thick with thoughts. It is up to us to choose which ones we allow entrance into our mind and which ones we reject. Some are obvious, some are much more subtle. Some are benign, some are very malignant, deadly if allowed to enter. The problem is that some of the most deadly thoughts are viewed in our society as acceptable, even if undesirable. We have allowed "political correctness" to dominate our choices in favor of Wisdom. And in this we are most foolish. We have chosen the attitude of "being fashionable" over being wise. I call this "accepted insanity."

For instance we accept disease as a legitimate experience, even though we hate experiencing it. Instead of rejecting the thought outright, realizing it can not be experienced unless we accept it, we embrace the horrid thought... unto our own destruction. Why do we do this? Because everyone does it. Everyone does it because we have been convinced that we have little to no choice, that we live under a "law" of chance and victim-hood. It is like being swept along a fast racing current and *not even realizing we can get out of the water* before we rush headlong over the waterfall only to crash into the rocks below.

I was giving a lecture to medical personal recently and when I got to the part that disease was a *learned experience* and we could reject it...and by doing so, not experience it...the look on their faces was incredulous. It would have been funny if the topic wasn't so serious to me. I told them they reminded me of what it must have been like for the townspeople the day Alexander Graham Bell told them they could talk into a box in their homes and people could hear them in their homes across town.

King David declares this Wisdom, "I would rather be a doorkeeper in the house of God than to sit at a banquet table with fools." (Psalm. 84:10) The "house of God" is our consciousness, our heart (in Bible terminology). To "be a doorkeeper" is to stand at the entrance to the door of our minds and determine what we allow in and what we won't. We do it for our physical homes, don't we? Why not at the place where we really live? To "sit at a table with fools," of course, is to eat whatever comes along with no regard for the value of the substance. This is *living randomly* as opposed to *living deliberately*. This is the difference between those who live in Wisdom and those who live in idle foolishness...which, of course, we have all done...and suffered the consequences. We will, after all, reap the harvest of what we sow.

You see words and thoughts are alive. They each have a frequency and travel in the atmosphere seeking a mind to rest upon. Unless we are made aware of this we will go through our lives not really thinking about what we are entertaining in our thought. It is an awakening indeed when we begin to be cognizant of this.

The Old Testament stories are so often about battles and wars, one wonders if that was all they did back then. But the deeper spiritual significance of this is clear. Each "enemy" that came to the Israelites in an attempt to overcome them *signified a thought* that if allowed would have utterly destroy them. To name a few, the Canannites mean division. The Perrizites mean strife. The Hivites mean fear and the Hittites mean hate. The Ammorites mean self love, while the Ammonites mean trusting in your own accomplishments to carry the day, instead of trusting in God. And so on. The list is endless as are the thoughts and ideologies we face unknowingly every day.

🫰 REBUILDING
THE WALL

The city of Jerusalem is symbolic of your consciousness. These nations (thoughts) were forever attempting to
scale the wall of defense to overtake the city. Often times
they did and the nation of Israel was decimated and scat-
tered throughout the world. The wall was built of stone
and the stones represent truths...absolute and eternal truths
that keep the destructive thoughts out of the city. The more
we fill our hearts and minds with truth, with the unchangeable, indestructible words of God, with the undeniable
knowledge of the true nature of God...the better our defense against invasion. Within the city was the temple and
within the temple was the dwelling place of the Glory and
strength of God, even as within our own being is the Light
and Glory of God. And just as the inhabitants of the city
were preoccupied with maintaining the wall of defense, so
must we be also. It is a discipline unlike any other, but
necessary for survival and peace.

When the nation became complacent and lazy in its
defense, it was overtaken by the Babylonian army and led
into captivity. The word Babylon means "the confusion of
many voices." This is "world thought" or mass mesmer-
ism, a tidal wave of hypnotic thought that captures the
world, unchallenged, and deadly in its consequences. The
common acceptance of disease, the many predictions of the
outcome of disease, the insane things we allow people to do
to our bodies... all in the name of acceptable treatments,
the myriads of "causes" of diseases, such as heredity, sea-

sonal changes, age, gender, contagious, etc., all this can be summed up as being enslaved or captured by Babylon.

Other accepted insanities which have enslaved mankind for generations is the religious belief that God *sent or caused* disease… to correct us, teach us, redirect us…punish us. That we need suffering to gain access to God and to His heavenly peace. All this deadly nonsense has made up the experience of being "held captive by Babylon." The result of accepting such ideologies is the sufferings, agonies and destruction we see all around us and within us.

We let the wall be torn down and the city be overcome. We fell asleep at the wall. Slowly the insidious ideas crept into our atmosphere of thought and without the truth to reject them, they took over the city. Now what do we do? We rebuild the wall. We replace the lies, the confusion with the unchangeable truth. For instance, if we realize we have been entertaining the idea that God might have allowed this for our good, we repent of that thought…reject it from our atmosphere of thought…and replace it with the realization that God does not punish, nor does He use evil to gain good. Our beliefs and subsequent attitudes invite the disasters we experience. Another way to put it is our sins punish us. It's good that they do. It enables us to clear them from our soul and allow the pure truth and Love that is God to rule and reign. Once we faithfully do this, the experience will naturally correct itself and we will find the healing or restoration we desire.

Every experience begins with thought. Not necessarily that you or anyone else consciously thought something into existence...but that we don't reject it for ourselves or others when the suggestion appears. And it appears from the general consciousness of the confusion of the world. This is important to understand. You didn't create this madness. You only failed to reject it for the knowledge of the truth when it appeared.

Thoughts come as suggestions. We are not required to accept them. We choose. Usually we choose by default, by not choosing anything at all. Soon we are accepting ideas for no other reason except they were spoken in our ears and found entrance into our consciousness. We must measure them against the absolute *truth of being*. What does that mean? It means we must look to what God says is the Eternal, unchangeable truth about Himself and about man, made in His image...and not look to what has been commonly accepted as the truth of life...or *our true being*. Even though the evidence is strong to the contrary, we must remember that *we are experiencing according to what we are believing.* When the basic belief is challenged and corrected, the experience will also correct itself. This is the law of reaping and sowing...or more popularly called the Law of attraction.

Jesus said that the Kingdom of Heaven... the authority of the truth and Presence of God... is within us and all around us. Paul said that "We live, move, and have *our being*" in this. It is as close as our beliefs. If we are not experiencing the goodness of this place and space, if we are not realizing the wonders of all that can be in our lives, we can begin to change this right now. It is "at hand." It is not far off, someplace to be realized at some later date. "*Today* if you will hear His voice, harden not your heart by unbelief." Goodness and fullness and wholeness and joy are part of being in the Kingdom of God, and it was eternally deemed that we be in this place continually, in consciousness and in reality. It is still, and always, available for us to enter in any time we choose. And it is not to be *earned*, as some say. It is done, it is finished, and it cannot be altered by man's ideas to the contrary.

Jesus said that the way to gain entrance into this realm of goodness, wholeness and completeness was to repent. To repent means to reject what has been accepted and to choose again. It is much more than simply being sorry for the choices we have made. We must choose differently.

Just *saying* truths will not do. We must kick the old thought out. We must reject it deliberately. There needs to be a moment when we say, "No, I reject this belief. I repent! I will now choose to believe something else. Even though up till now I have chosen to believe according to world thought... I have chosen to believe according to physical evidence... I have believed what I *saw* rather than what is *Eternally true*. Now I choose to choose differently!"

Not realizing that we are *seeing what we are believing*, we thought we were believing what we saw...but not so! We see what we believe is true. If we are willing to correct what we are believing, we will find that we *see differently* as well. This is how healings really happen. We believe truth instead of evidence! We choose to believe what God says is true in spite of what is seen or felt. And when we do this, the feelings will follow. The experience will follow. This is what Jesus meant by "repent." Start over. Eject the old thought, the believed suggestion. Rebuild the wall. How do we do that? After we reject the old, we fill our minds, our hearts, our minutes, hours and days with what is eternally true.

Read materials that focus solely upon the absolute truth. Nothing watered down will do. Read, study and pray. Remember that we possess the Mind of God. Whatever is true for your particular situation will be spoken deep in your heart. When it is, speak it out loud. Let your words testify to the truth you know.

Always and only speak the truth. If you are in a situation where others are speaking error, thereby glorifying it once again, simply hold your peace. Don't try to convince them of your understanding. They will deny it, and attempt to convince you that what you are seeing and experiencing is the only possible truth and they will say you are denying the obvious. They will not understand.

I remember when my second daughter was born with so many pulmonary problems and was not expected to live, they asked me if they could simply stop all efforts and just let her die. Medically I understood their position, I had been there many times myself with parents. But when I said "no!" they sent a psychiatrist in to tell me that I was "in denial." To those who have never reached for faith with all their hearts, to those who have never known the true nature of man, forever in the image of God, and to those who deny such truths in favor of "their reality"…it certainly would be absurd to hear us speak of such things. So there is nothing to gain by getting into an argument with darkness and confusion. It only serves as a temptation to drag you into it once again. Protect your space!

Nehemiah was an Israelite during the time of the captivity of Babylon, just as we are now. His heart longed to live once again in his beloved Jerusalem (city of peace) but the city was destroyed and the wall was decimated. He returned to the place where Jerusalem once stood and gathered like-minded souls, also from the captivity, to rebuild the wall that the city might once again be inhabited. If you read this very short book in the Old Testament, you will find that they met with certain adversaries determined to squash their efforts. These men finally sought to kill them in order to stop them. But Nehemiah was full of the Spirit of God and Wisdom prevailed. At one point he told them that he was no longer going to answer them because they "had no part in this matter." And so it is with us.

Another story found in Isaiah, chapters 36 and 37, was similar, but the wall was already built and the city flourished under the government of the mercy and goodness of God. This is the time when Hezekiah was king of Israel. The day came when the armies of the Assyrians surrounded the city and declared they were going to tear down the wall and enter the city to once again take the inhabitants captive. The fear of the invading Assyrians was strong throughout the land because they had overcome every standing city that they ever decided to destroy. Assyria might be symbolic of the accepted intelligence of the land. That which is declared and accepted to be true. And, as such, their words were feared. Surely what they said would come to pass! They told them two things that almost tore the hearts of the people in half. First they told them that God had sent them (the Assyrians) to destroy them (the Israelites) for their many sins (ever heard that one?)

Then they told them to "look around" and see that every nation who ever tried to stop them failed. They had the power and the evidence to prove it. Faced with destruction in our lives of any sort, we fail to heal when we look at how others have faired in the same circumstance. In this there is no Wisdom! Look only to God. Look only to what you know is absolute truth. "Look not to the left or to the right." But look straight ahead. Hezekiah, in his Wisdom told his people, "Answer them not a word!" No matter what was said, the Wisdom remained, "Answer them not a word."

To "resist evil" is to declare that you yet see it as a power to destroy. If you hold your peace, God will answer them for you. And so He did. Soon the entire Assyrian army had destroyed each other and the city was spared.

Many such stories we read in the Old testament, all sharing with us the way to arise in victory over any and every appearance of evil...no matter how obtrusive it may appear...or who believes what about it!

CONCLUSION

Many ideas have been discussed here and my hope and prayer is that they carry each reader to the healing and safety they require. If you find yourself full of ideas but not sure how to proceed to utilize them, just pause and ask. If you are unsure of whatever you have read or understood, just ask. If anything I have said here ran headlong into already held beliefs and ideologies and you found it disturbing, just stop and ask the Holy Spirit to sort it all out for you. The purpose of this wonderful gift of the Spirit of Jesus Christ sent into our hearts was just that…to lead and guide us into the wholeness that we seek, to grow and mature us into the manifestation of the sons of God that we are. If you are faithful to humbly ask, you will always receive an answer. It will appear to you in a way that you will be able to understand and accept it.

Remember that the whole Divine Intention for us being here is that the Life of the Eternal One may be revealed in, to and through us. "It is your Father's good pleasure to give you the Kingdom." Just ask.

REFERENCES

John 15: 7,16